D1431298

The Sun Will Rise

*A Story of Rising Again
After Unimaginable Loss*

NATALIE SCOTT

WESTBOW
PRESS®
A DIVISION OF THOMAS NELSON
& ZONDERVAN

WestBow Press books may be ordered through booksellers or by contacting:

WestBow Press
A Division of Thomas Nelson & Zondervan
1663 Liberty Drive
Bloomington, IN 47403
www.westbowpress.com
1 (866) 928-1240

ISBN: 978-1-9736-6487-1 (sc)
ISBN: 978-1-9736-6489-5 (hc)
ISBN: 978-1-9736-6488-8 (e)

Library of Congress Control Number: 2019907182

Print information available on the last page.

WestBow Press rev. date: 06/14/2019

Dedication

Dedicated with all my love to my baby girl, Eleanora Lynn Scott and to her brothers and my rainbow babies, Pierce and Everett. Mommy loves you all more than words can describe.

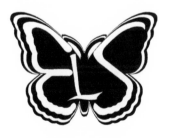

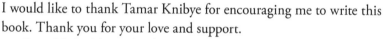

I would like to thank Tamar Knibye for encouraging me to write this book. Thank you for your love and support.

I would also like to thank Nina Lichtenstein for taking her precious time to help edit the book. Your time and insight mean a lot to me.

To my mom, thank you for always believing in every dream I have ever had. Thank you for knowing I should be a writer long before I knew it myself. Thank you for everything you did from the second Eleanora left us to join her Pop Pop in heaven and her Heavenly Father. We could not have done it without you.

To Pierce and Everett, thank you for loving me so fiercely even though I am broken. Thank you for holding me up when I have had no strength to stand. For encouraging me with the innocence of a child. Thank you for telling everyone you have a sister. She will live on in both of you. Thank you for all you are and all you do.

Lastly, I would like to thank my husband, Nick, for walking this journey with me. It has not been an easy road for either of us but we have weathered it together. Thank you for letting me have the time and space to cry freely, to shout when I needed to shout, to fall apart and know you are standing there to support me and for loving me through the storm. Thank you for laughing with me when all we both wanted to do was cry. Thank you for inside jokes no one could possibly ever understand. Thank you for believing I would one day write this book. I love you and know no one could love me back quite the way you do. Come What May!

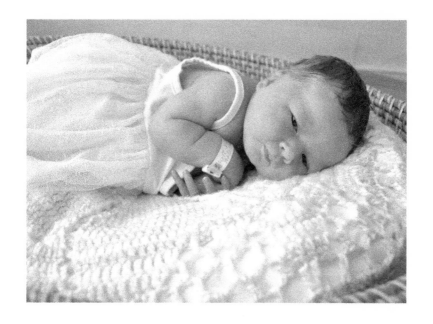

Eleanora Lynn Scott
June 17-22, 2011

"I'll love you forever,
I'll like you for always,
As long as I am living
My baby you'll be."

Love You Forever by Robert Munsch

Preface

I wanted to write this book for a long time, but I could never think of what the end result would be. In my profession as a writer, I have a goal in mind. This article will be for Camp and that one for my organization's upcoming event. I could not come up with the purpose for this book. My friend encouraged me to just sit down and start writing and with that push I did. I sat down one day and started the story. I cried over the keyboard most days I wrote. I felt the pain all over again. I lived the moments breath by breath, heartbeat by pounding heartbeat. I wrote through tears and shaking fingers. I wrote through my fears of failure. I just wrote. I still had no clear vision of the end result.

One day while cutting potatoes, I was having a conversation with God in my head. He often visits there and quietly waits for me to sit down with Him. I asked Him what the purpose was for the book. I asked Him for help with the direction. In response I heard Him say, "I have been waiting. I thought you'd never ask." So, to God I give all the glory for guidance and for loving me when I told Him to just go away. For bringing me to this place of peace that I never felt I would reach after years of living in blackness. For being my Daddy and wrapping His arms around me when I needed Him the most. And for not turning His back on me, never leaving my side. Thank you.

This book has been a labor of love. It is my heart and soul revealed to the world. It makes me feel exposed and vulnerable. Yet here I stand on the precipice ready to leap.

Part 1

My Story

Chapter 1

The Beginning

How do you begin writing about the end? Where does the story start? Does it really end?

This is my story. Or should I say, the story of my sweet Eleanora.

The journey with Eleanora really started on my 27th birthday, long before she was born or even conceived. Nick and I had been married for almost two years with the idea of kids somewhere in the future, but not anytime soon. After being laid off and searching for a job for a year, Nick finally found one and started in November. Swinging 12 hour shifts and traveling 1.5 hours each way was tough, but it was a job and it was a good one.

My birthday in January went like every other year with no one making a big deal, but one major thing happened. When I woke up that day something clicked for me. That morning I knew with absolute certainty that I was ready for a baby. Nick didn't understand and I can't really explain it either, but I knew whenever it happened, I was ready.

Typing it out now, it seems silly. With all of the uphill battles we were already facing, I can't explain why, except that I felt it in my heart. I told him it did not need to be today or tomorrow or even next month, but I wanted to start the conversation. While most of our relationship we were on the same page, we were both ready to move in with each other, get engaged and married – we hit a road block when it came to the topic of a baby. At one point, about a month after telling him I was ready, he told me he did not think he ever wanted kids. I told him that was a deal breaker. The conversation stopped there and we went out that night.

Fast forward to June, I had a major medical issue and Nick was so afraid he was going to lose me. I was in pretty bad shape when one day he turned to me and said, "I am ready now, let's have a baby." I laughed because at that time my body was not ready. It took two more months and we started officially trying.

Looking at every app and website I could get my hands on, I figured out when I would ovulate and we tried and tried. Well, it turns out my body is not predictable. We would have never gotten pregnant if I had relied solely on those apps. I had a 40-day cycle that was not consistent. So, it did not happen that first month. We had to wait another 40 days to test. I always wonder, if it had been that first egg or that sperm, would I be sitting here today telling my story? If it had happened that first month that baby would not be Eleanora. That's the way life works. I will never know.

The next round, we threw all the apps out the window. I still charted everything just in case, but my body was erratic so the chart did not make any sense. Against all odds, that second round trying every other day between a swinging schedule for 40 days, two pink lines appeared. Those lines were just the beginning of a forever journey that has changed our lives.

It took eight months for Nick to be ready and two more months of trying to get pregnant with Eleanora. Ten months, the same amount of time it takes to grow a baby in your womb. It took ten more months to grow her into the beautiful baby we met on June 17. She was only with us on earth for 5 days. It took one second for me to fall in love with her; before I knew her foot in my ribs, knew the rhythm of her movements, before I knew her sex or her name and before I knew her face. I will spend a lifetime loving her and a lifetime living with a hole in my heart that only my baby girl can fill.

We had a perfect pregnancy. I follow that by saying I was sick as a dog for the first 16 weeks. I could not keep anything down and was nauseated all day long. My boss even told me to stay home one day because I looked green. After that all was well. I started gaining weight and watched in awe as my belly, once flat, grew a little bump and then a bigger swell. I felt the first flutters about the time my nausea ended. Each movement was a welcome reminder of the precious gift I was growing. I was doing an amazing thing and could not be happier.

As we inched closer and closer to my due date, our joy and excitement grew. I was due on June 30th, but was told in the middle of May that she would be here no later than two to three weeks. That was the only appointment Nick missed. My brother, Robert, went with me. I told him the news first that Eleanora would be there in two to three weeks. He patiently listened to the same details as I repeated them to Nick and my mom. I can still remember how it felt that day knowing she was coming sooner rather than later.

Chapter 2

It's TIME!

"It's time!" The excitement was building. She is coming tonight. Or so we thought. Two times we went to maternity in hopes of meeting our much-anticipated baby girl. Two times we were sent home, the nurses saying I was in the beginning stages of labor and that I should return later that night further along in my labor. Two times the contractions stopped in the middle of the night. I sigh just thinking about how stubborn everyone thought she was. Now I wonder if she didn't want to come out because she knew what would happen when she did. Thankfully I will get to ask her one day.

When it really was time, it wasn't what we pictured. There was no rushing to triage, contracting all the way. It wasn't like in the movies with the wife yelling at the husband to hurry up. It was not like that at all.

I was induced in the early morning hours at 38 weeks because of all the false alarms and a horrible pregnancy rash that was spreading all over my body. As we counted down the hours and watched morning turn into afternoon, evening, and night, I started to realize that she was not coming that day. She wanted to make an entrance and she wanted it to be on her own terms.

As easy as my pregnancy was, my labor was the complete opposite. The epidural did its job at the beginning, but sometime in the afternoon it stopped working. By the time I delivered Eleanora, I was practically doing it naturally. I was in agony despite getting the pain medicine to avoid this. I felt everything during her delivery, a blessing and a curse.

After 17 hours of labor she came in the early hours of the following morning at 12:45 a.m. after three hours of pushing. She was, without exaggeration, the most beautiful child ever to be born, ever to exist in this world. She had the face of an angel. I remember looking at her in awe. I spent 10 months imagining what she would look like and my best image could not compare to this perfection. She was 7 pounds 13 ounces and 21 inches long.

We named her Eleanora Lynn. Her name was picked long before she was born, but it was a struggle agreeing on the perfect name that fit her and we both liked. Many names were texted back and forth. So many were turned down. When I came up with the name Eleanor I thought Nick would hate it, but surprisingly he fell in love. We would nickname her Ellie when she was small, but I worried about what her name would become as she got older and outgrew Ellie.

When I was looking up the meaning of Eleanor, I saw the name Eleanora and that felt like a better fit for the baby growing inside of me. Ellie when she was small and Nora when she grew up. The irony of me picking a forever name for her is not lost on me. Her name means light or mercy, which I still feel is so fitting for her.

For 10 months, I feared losing her. I could not have been so lucky to have gotten everything I ever wanted on the first try. I waited and waited for her to be taken away and now she was here. I had her in my arms and I was never letting her go. When I heard her cry for the first time I let out the biggest sigh of relief. Now that she was here, nothing could take her away.

I was elated. On top of the moon? Yes, that was me dancing in delight. When my mom and mother-in-law visited in those very early hours they kept saying, "There is no way you just had a baby, you look amazing!" I thought, look at what I made. Look at what I brought into this world! I did it! I could not stop smiling. She is here!

My mom told me later that when she first met Eleanora, she looked at her face and thought she was staring at an angel. Her face was too perfect.

Her first night we had to stay in labor and delivery since every other person on the floor had come and gone with their baby. I had listened to screams of labor pain, crying babies and squeals of delight for 17 hours. There were no rooms left on the maternity floor for our brand-new family. I didn't mind. I had my girl. I remember waking up and looking over at her in amazement through the clear bassinet. She was real! I just kept staring at her in disbelief. She was here. She was alive. She was perfect. She was mine!!! The nurses were crazy about her. I beamed with pride.

Later that morning we moved to a maternity room. Over the course of the next two days friends and family showed up to meet my little girl. She was the first grandchild. She was loved and wanted so much by so many people. They ooed and ahhed over her.

My friend, Shelagh, was afraid to pick her up because she was so tiny. She asked me to unwrap her and once she saw Eleanora's chubby little legs she snatched her up. I remember the pure joy and elation on Shelagh's face rocking this baby she had waited so long to hold.

I had three separate surprise baby showers. For someone who is not used to being in the spotlight, I was in heaven. All this love for my little girl! How lucky can we be? Her closet was filled with all of her clothes waiting to be worn, clothes that so many times I ran my fingers along smiling, as I imagined watching her grow from newborn to three months and so on. Hues of pink, purple, yellow, green, and white filled her closet. Her room, comprised of an antique white crib, changing table/dresser and wardrobe cast against purple painted walls and bumble bees fluttering about glowed with the excitement we felt.

Her rocking chair that I eagerly sat in with growing anticipation to match my growing belly, was motionless in the corner waiting for late night feedings and cuddles. Her dresser was filled with onesies that were folded to perfection, frilly socks, hair bows, burp cloths, receiving blankets, and toys. There was no denying she was wanted and loved.

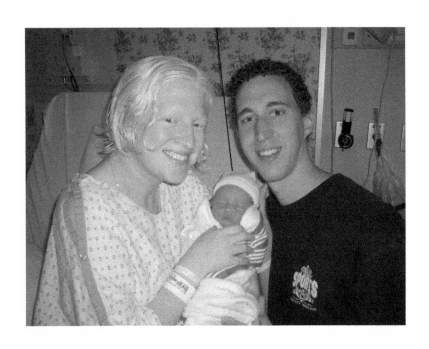

Chapter 3

You Are All I Need

The next day, the day we were set to go home for the first time as three, was Father's Day. What a lucky man, my husband, for I could not have given him a greater gift than that of our sweet Eleanora. She was everything we ever wanted. While he packed the car, I dressed my sweet little baby up in a pale peach dress. I wanted everything to be perfect when we brought her home so I searched high and low for the perfect dress. In fact, my mom and I drove an hour to pick it up since it was unavailable at the store near us.

Eleanora, my little trooper, did not mind being dressed up at all. I put a sweater and hat set on her that my mom made. I had to roll up the sleeves because it was too big for our little sweetheart. I laughed and cooed at her and she just went with the flow. I took a million pictures, hat on, hat off, sweater on and off. I took pictures of her little white shoes and socks. Some with a pacifier and some without. Then we were ready.

They wheeled me down to the car as I glowed with pride. Eleanora was wrapped in a colorful round blanket made by my mom. I felt like I was on top of the world! There has never been a moment before or since that I was ever this happy and serene. Life was perfect.

Too afraid to leave her for even a moment, I road in the backseat with her on the drive home. Once home, we changed her into a more sensible sleeper outfit with butterflies and caterpillars on it. Her daddy excitedly gave her a tour of the house, then I took Eleanora to her bedroom to nurse her. I had been struggling on and off to latch Eleanora properly in the hospital, but once I settled into the rocker in her room, she latched on perfectly and nursed for 45 minutes. She was amazing. What a beautiful gift.

My mom came over with sushi and gladly held her granddaughter nearby while we ate. Then my mom left and it was just our little family of three.

Eleanora did have jaundice the last day in the hospital and was required to spend several hours receiving phototherapy, or what we call "under the blue lights." She donned cute little "sunglasses" to protect her eyes from the light. On Monday, the day after we arrived home, I noticed Eleanora looked a little more yellow and felt there was reason to be concerned. We called the doctor and they had us come in. The doctor said she looked okay, but sent us for bloodwork at the hospital just in case. He also told me that certain fabrics or colors in a room might make her look more yellow. If I was worried, I should change the environment and see if that helped since it might just be a reflection. The bloodwork was fine and we went about our merry way.

The doctor told us it would be a good idea to put Eleanora in the sun to help with jaundice. He said it may not help much, but every little bit makes a difference. I put her in the swing next to the sliding glass doors. Nick and I sat near her on the couches and at one point, I said how much I miss her. He looked at me like I had 10 heads. How could I miss her when she was right in front of us? Aside from family and friends holding her, I had not been "away" from her for 10 months.

Even though we were in the same room, I missed the feel of her in my arms.

Shortly afterwards, I walked away for just a second when Nick called me in because she was sucking her thumb for the first time. He said he's never seen me move so fast. Camera in hand, I snapped the cutest pictures capturing her with her thumb in her mouth and fingers in her eyes. She was squinting up at us with one eye open wondering what all the fuss was about.

The next morning, I rocked and nursed Eleanora. She seemed to nurse really well if I walked around. As I was holding her after nursing, something suddenly felt terribly wrong. Very calmly, because I did not want to alarm her, I placed her sleepy head in her swing and ran to the bathroom.

I yanked down my pants and a blood clot the size of a grapefruit fell out. I was told that if anything larger than a quarter came out, I was to rush immediately to the hospital because I could be hemorrhaging. I was afraid to run up the stairs to get my still sleeping husband so I called his name and banged on the steps to indicate he should hurry. We rushed to the hospital maternity ward. Thankfully, I was allowed to keep Eleanora with me since I was nursing her. After a checkup, we were cleared to go home. They made it seem like we were crazy for even coming in. That afternoon we said no more hospitals for a long time! Poor Eleanora had gone to the hospital every day of her life.

In the wee hours of the next morning I was trying desperately to get Eleanora to latch properly. She was frustrated and crying hysterically. I told her in that moment that she was it for me. I would never have another baby because I wouldn't want another baby's cries to wake her up in the middle of the night. She was all I ever needed.

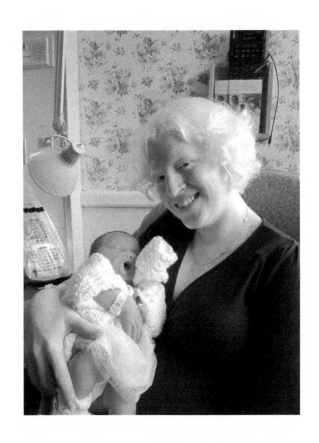

Chapter 4

Endless Night

Though he brings grief, he also shows compassion because of the greatness of his unfailing love. For he does not enjoy hurting people or causing them sorrow.

Lamentations 3:32-33 (NLT)

I continued to struggle to always properly latch Eleanora without a lot of frustration on her part and a lot of the feeling of failure on my part. I did not give up though. The next morning, I was thrilled when she latched on and ate beautifully.

Afterwards, I just held her looking at her perfect, angelic face. I looked down at her resting face and looked up briefly at something on the TV. When I looked back down I knew something was not right. She looked yellow again, but in my mind a different shade of yellow than two days before. I did what the doctor said. Trying not to panic, I took her into the kitchen. She looked the same. I asked my husband if she looked yellow and he said she did look a little more yellow. I knew in my gut something was not right. There was no science backing up my suspicions, just a motherly instinct.

We took the mommy classes at the hospital to be completely prepared for both labor and after the baby was born. We used this knowledge to help assess the situation. Aside from a voice screaming in my head, there was no need for panic. We called the doctor again and told them she was yellow and something did not feel right, not with her, but emotionally. Again, they had us come in.

We rushed to the office and waited in the waiting room for what felt like hours. I wanted to scream that something was wrong, but again it was just my heart saying it. I kept asking my husband, is she breathing? Yes. Is her heart still beating? Yes. I started crying in the waiting room. He told me to stop. I said I couldn't help it that I knew something was wrong. He told me I was being ridiculous. When we were finally seen I started undressing her in the room.

When the doctor came in, he saw something we did not and started CPR. Still to this day I don't know what he saw. She was not blue and her lips were not blue. She would even pull her eyes shut if we tried to open them. He yelled to call 911 and that is when my life fell apart. We were pulled from the room. They kept working on her. I felt so helpless and stupid for not knowing.

The staff tried to comfort us with encouraging words. I remember at one point I was standing at the door of the building waiting for her to come out and wondering what was taking so long. Then we were pulled into a room with another doctor in the practice, a very kind doctor who had been Eleanora's doctor while she was in the hospital. I kept asking her if Eleanora would be okay. She kept saying the other doctor was breathing for Eleanora. Surely, they could bring her back I thought against all reason. I was just holding a happy, healthy baby one minute and, what felt like the next minute, doctors were fighting for her next breath. It all happened in an instant.

They put Eleanora on a stretcher, making her tiny body look even smaller. Her pediatrician put his hand on my shoulder and said, "This is Mom." It is an odd thing to remember, but it made me feel special. Yes, I am her mom. She is mine. When I went to climb in the ambulance like I have seen so many people on television do, they told me to go sit up front so they could continue to work on her. I guess I should have known then that it was not a good sign, but I was not ready to give up.

Before we started driving, the driver asked if there were any changes. I didn't hear the response. I called my mom and she was already on her way. Nick had called and was following us in our car with an empty car seat where Eleanora should have been.

The ambulance never turned on the siren. My mom, on the phone, asked why she couldn't hear the sirens. I asked in a shaking voice why there were no sirens. The driver did not answer. Having no communication with me, Nick was becoming increasingly frustrated as he navigated the streets behind the ambulance, which did not appear to be in a rush at all. For part of the trip we had a police escort blocking all of the roadways, but then we were on our own. Nick did not have trouble keeping up.

When we got to the hospital, I jumped out of the ambulance ready to run into the emergency room after Eleanora. I can still hear the sound of Nick's sandals hitting the pavement as he ran to be by our side. "Why didn't he turn on the sirens?" was the first thing he said. We were ushered into an emergency room where a team of doctors and nurses were ready to save our sweet baby girl.

We watched and listened as they tried one thing after another. They had her heart beating again, but they were helping it along. I prayed nonstop the entire time. I prayed for a miracle. I believe in miracles and was hoping that this day we would witness one.

Nick and I had a nurse, a pediatrician, and a social worker standing by our side. The nurse was very kind, letting us know each step of the process. She seemed to read our emotions and know when to reassure us. There was so much beeping and movement, but no answers. At one point it became too much. I ran from the room, sat on the floor, and started crying hysterically. I felt like I couldn't breathe. Nick followed me out. So did the social worker. They called for a wheelchair because I wasn't allowed to sit on the floor. I told them I did not need a wheelchair and regained my composure to a certain degree knowing that I had to be strong for my baby. I went back into the room only to confront the same flurried movements and nonstop beeping noises.

For a moment, everyone stopped what they were doing. I looked at the nurse, my eyes pleading for answers. She said they wanted to see if Eleanora could breathe on her own and if her heart would beat without help. The room was silent as her steady beat only fluttered without assistance. The activity picked up again as the doctors tried various strategies. One doctor kept asking, "Does anyone have any ideas?" They had ideas. They exhausted them all. Then they stopped. They called her time of death. And that was the end of my world.

As they wrapped Eleanora up and placed a pink hat on her head, the lead doctor informed us that they had tried everything. He told us she was gone in a cold, unfeeling manner. I asked if they could try anything else and he replied, "Just think about her quality of life." I understand that the ER must harden the staff, but I often wonder if that doctor ever quietly mourns for babies lost like mine.

I asked if they could keep trying. How was I supposed to go on living without my baby girl? How could the Earth keep spinning when her life had just ended and so had mine? In that moment, I wanted to lie down with her and stop breathing. If it were that easy I would not be here writing her story. I would have avoided the pain and emptiness that lay in wait. I would have said goodbye to the cruelty of life. I would not have gone on without her, but that choice was not up to me.

They put me on her hospital bed and I held her while crying and continuing to pray. My mom and mother-in-law were waiting in the grieving room. The head doctor had given them the horrific news in a very matter of fact way. It is his job. He sees death every day. I don't blame him.

When they both came in to see me, I looked at my mom, who knows all of the many difficulties I have had to overcome and survive, and asked her point blank "Why does God hate me?" For me, it seemed the only logical conclusion as to why God would do this to us. I have since made peace with the fact that God did not kill my child. The way I view it now is that He was weeping with me. That just like an earthly father, my Father in heaven was hurting for me and feeling the sting of the pain coursing through my body. The image in my head is that His arms were wrapped around our little family, soaking up the tears flowing from our eyes. God is not evil. This was not a way to punish me. I can say that now, but it has been a long road to discovery and realization.

Psalm 56:8 (NLT)

You keep track of all my sorrows. You have collected all my tears in your bottle. You have recorded each one in your book.

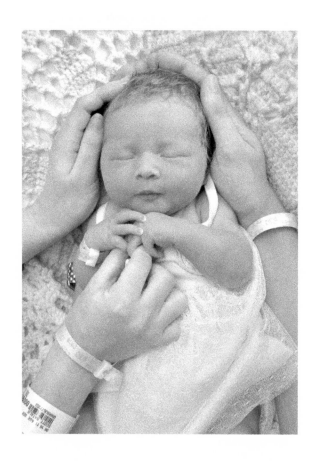

Chapter 5

Searching for Answers

We did absolutely nothing to harm or hurt our baby, but the next series of events exemplifies the ills of society. I was asked to leave Eleanora in the emergency room for just a moment while the police asked us questions. This seemed fairly normal, albeit painful to leave her after I had her in my arms again. My husband, baby, and I were all separated. Nick and I were each questioned by two different officers in two different rooms to make sure there was no foul play. Meanwhile, every cop in the area was searching my home. My brothers offered to let them into the house, otherwise they would have kicked down the door. They rushed to my house with the key.

The officers searched high and low and found nothing. My brothers tried their best to be patient while the cops searched my house, but they could not help but feel overprotective for their innocent sister who had just lost her baby. I was later told the cops asked some odd questions, such as where all of Eleanora's clothes were kept. My younger brother stared at them baffled and said, "My sister got so many clothes for the baby, she had to return some. They are in the closet where they belong." When the cops opened the door, they would have seen a closet full of her clothes, all hung up perfectly in order from newborn to 24 months. The stylish clothes from us, friends and family were a physical representation of the excitement to welcome a new baby into the world. She even had a flower girl dress ready to be worn at her Uncle's wedding in the fall. No clothes? Certainly not this little girl.

If they opened her drawers, they would have seen perfectly folded and stacked onesies, frilly socks, hair bows, receiving blankets, and burp cloths. Her wardrobe, a very feminine piece with an oval mirror, in front of which she could one day play dress up, was filled with books, shampoos, and baby powder. What they would have found was a crib with sheets containing a bee pattern to match the bees buzzing about on her purple walls. Foul play? No. Just a screaming house with the echoes of a cooing baby now gone. Yes, that is indeed what they found. The house we abandoned that morning as we rushed to the doctor was nothing but ready for a lifetime of happiness.

After we were questioned, we went to the grieving room. It is all a little hazy now, but I remember simple acts of kindness. My younger brother couldn't get close to me because my mother-in-law and her boyfriend were hugging me and Nick, so he grabbed my hand. He held it, rubbing it softly. I caught his eye and I know his heart was broken too. He did not say a word, but he did not let go of my hand.

After the cops finished their investigation, we were cleared of any possible wrongdoing. We went into a small room with a stark, cold metal bed, the same one my stepdad laid on five years before. My stepdad, a 53-year-old man filled the table. Despite his young age at time of death, it made more sense for him to have laid there than for my five-day-old baby, who had barely made a ripple in the sea of life.

At first, we were told that we were not allowed to pick her up. I stood over her whispering how much I love her and kissing her sweet face. Eventually someone said something that led the officers standing guard to inform me that of course I could pick her up. She looked so perfect. Take away the backdrop of a cold, unfeeling, hospital room and I was just a mommy holding her newborn baby girl.

I rocked her and cried over her. I took her little pink hat off and ran my fingers through her perfectly highlighted blonde hair. I never put a hat on her so she didn't look like herself with it on. Knowing I would never see her pretty, soft hair again, I soaked in every moment, committing it to memory. I caressed her hair and kissed her cheeks trying to memorize everything about her. I wanted to create a permanent map of her in my heart. I breathed her in, hoping to fill my lungs forever with her precious scent.

A hospital pastor, I assumed that's what she was, asked if we would like to baptize her and we gratefully said yes. So, with our family surrounding us, we had the only celebration or milestone Eleanora would ever have. She did not make it to a week or month old. We would never gather around a cake and sing happy birthday to a bubbling one-year-old. We would never see her hold her head up for the first time, roll over, sit up, stand, or walk. We were robbed of it all. But in this moment at least, we could pause and celebrate her. Her spirit was already gone far away to heaven, but we baptized her earthly body that day. About a week later, we received an envelope commemorating this day of her life. We keep it amongst her things and I smile when I see it. I am so glad this service was available to us.

I don't remember the words that were said during her baptism, but it is as though a pause button was pressed. For a moment, we were no longer saying good bye, but stopping to bless a life lived. The pastor was tender and respectful and did not treat us like we were holding a forever sleeping baby. Now that the wound is not so fresh, I look back on those moments and cherish them. The pastor cut some of her hair and put it in a little keepsake for us. I often look at her hair and let the waves of emotion sweep over me.

It felt like each moment moving forward was harder than the last. A prayer was said over baby Eleanora and then came the impossible, letting go. How do you kiss your baby knowing it will be the last time? How do you give the final hug and snuggle? How do you walk away knowing your heart is being left behind? How do you go on with life? Leaving her there in that cold, empty room devoid of feelings and emotions was indescribably soul crushing. It was nothing less than impossible. I was put in a wheelchair and pushed out to the car. In what felt like a cruel, insensitive joke, the sun was shining on a beautifully warm June day. Oh, how the weather was a juxtaposition to the storm raging in my body, mind, and heart.

My brother-in-law pulled the car up and Nick quickly removed the car seat base from the center of the back seat. The yellow, gray, white, and black patterned car seat matched her bees in her room, the stroller and the diaper bag. It had been installed and inspected by the car seat safety person at the DMV. We did everything in our power to ensure Eleanora's safety in this world before she was born. Now the car seat was quickly removed and put in the back of the car to make room for me and Nick in the back seat.

We had rushed to the hospital in hopes of saving Eleanora. Now there was no rush. There was just emptiness. Empty car seat. Empty back seat. Empty room. Empty home. Emptiness in my soul.

Everything felt wrong. I waited so long to have Eleanora. She was so perfect. She was my dream come true. And now we were in the back seat of our car driving away with nothing but broken hearts and shattered dreams. I was a hollowed-out shell of a person having left all that I am in the hospital room with my baby. None of this was right.

Chapter 6

Empty Cradle, Broken Heart

This chapter is named after a book by Deborah Davis, Ph.D. given to me by my friend Danielle after Eleanora passed away.

When we got home, all I wanted to do was wander around aimlessly, but there were so many people there. Everyone was trying to help. How could anyone help? My miracle was gone. My mom called the doctor to get medicine to ease my mind, but I refused to take it. Why put off the pain until tomorrow? I wanted to hurt. I felt like it was my fault she was gone. I am her mommy. It was my job to protect her from this world and I failed. I failed so miserably. Why did I deserve to escape the pain? I felt that I deserved every bit of pain the emptiness could inflict and still it would never match the punishment I felt I deserved. I turned down the medicine. To this day, I am glad that I did.

My mom's boss kindly sent food to feed all the family members that had gathered at the house. I couldn't eat. Why should I? I was no longer eating for two because my beautiful girl was not here. Why bother? Everyone ate and talked. My mind was elsewhere. My mom asked if she could call the funeral home. The question ripped my heart out because the funeral home only served to emphasize that Eleanora was never coming back. She calmly told me that they would go get her from the hospital so she was not laying there alone. She called and made the arrangements.

My mom sensed I needed a break from everyone and sent me upstairs to lie down. However, first she sent my brother up to move the bassinet from my bedside to Eleanora's room. I laid in the dark, alone, my breasts full and aching to feed my little one. Meanwhile, my mom sent everyone home.

I heard a quiet knock on the door. It was my friend Danielle. She was in the middle of buying a car when she heard the news. She dropped everything and rushed to my house. She walked out of the car dealership right in the middle of the deal to be by my side. You might say she is crazy, but she is a fellow loss mom. She lost her daughter, Mikayla, a couple of years before I lost Eleanora. She knows all too well the pain of losing a child. She hugged me, listened to me cry, and sat quietly by my side.

I asked her how one goes on to have any more kids since she had another son after she lost Mikayla. She smiled and replied, "You go into labor at 30 weeks, have your baby at 33 weeks and call that baby Michael." That was her experience anyway. Life does go on. Your baby is never replaced and life is never, ever the same.

Danielle left. My mom came up and checked on me. She tucked me in like she did when I was a little girl. How helpless she must have felt as a mother who could not kiss this pain away, like she did with all the scrapes when I was a child.

After everyone left and the house was quiet, the silence became deafening. It is hard to describe, but it felt like the sound of a thousand people shrieking around me all at once, closing in on me and choking the breath from my lungs. Nick and I decided to walk around the neighborhood to escape.

We barely made it out the front door when our neighbor approached us, excited about the new baby. She, like the rest of the neighbors, saw the pink balloons and sign go up to announce Eleanora was here. She was the first of many people I would have to tell that Eleanora was in heaven. It shook her to the core. She was left speechless with nothing to do but embrace me in a hug. This reaction of shock and an inability to know what to say comes as no surprise now. What does one say when this happens? Sudden death defies the promise of life bestowed upon babies at birth.

With an awkward goodbye, we continued walking until it was dark outside. When we returned home with heavy hearts, the silence was no less suffocating.

Nick was able to sleep that night and every night. My night was filled with wakefulness and bad dreams. I dreamt I was holding Eleanora again, but not without the reality of my current situation. In my dream I was holding Eleanora, wrapped in a blanket, but she was blue. When I awoke with a start, I was not holding Eleanora, but rather I was clinging tightly to a pillow, holding on desperately. When I glanced over to where Eleanora was sleeping so peacefully just the night before, I was reminded that it was not just a bad dream. She was gone. Her bassinet was gone. My hopes and dreams for her and our family were gone.

I wondered how Nick could sleep. How he could snore through the night and wake late in the morning. Despite a nearly sleepless night, I still arose early with nothing to do. If yesterday was the last day of my world as I knew it before it came crashing down all around me, then today was day one of my new life. Day one of the rest of my life walking, breathing and living with a gaping hole in my heart. How would I put one foot in front of the other?

Chapter 7

Diapers to Flowers

In the first few days of my "new normal" I was kept busy by things I never expected to be doing. Days of nursing, changing diapers, and sitting quietly with a snoozing baby were abruptly replaced with funeral arrangements, flowers and other similarly unfathomable tasks.

The man from the funeral home was kind enough to visit my home rather than making me go there. I attended this meeting in my pajamas, which consisted of Nick's old shirt that once upon a time smelled like him and Nick's old oversized pants – crotch opening included.

Unlike the doctor, the man from the funeral home was gentle and caring. He'd never walked this path personally, but his manner was soothing. He guided us through the process and let us pause when we needed a minute. When he offered us the two options for "caskets" for Eleanora's funeral service, I was in shock. To me, they looked like dressed up shoe boxes and there was no way my baby girl was going to be seen in a shoe box.

For many people, this would be their first time meeting Eleanora. For everyone, this would be the last time they ever saw her. She deserved better. Where I could not fulfill my role as a mommy to save her life, the very least I could do was be her advocate in death. When I suggested her bassinet be used instead, he happily agreed. He even offered to come pick it up for us.

Shelagh, who had been with me through the whole pregnancy, as well as there the day Eleanora was born, told my mom she would not come until I was ready for her. Everything that had happened thus far seemed too much for her to bear, but nonetheless she arrived just as the man from the funeral home was packing up. My mom led her to the family room so I could finish the preparations for Eleanora's service. As soon as she saw me, she burst into tears, hugged me with all her might and said, "I am so sorry." Shelagh is not known to cry or to hug, but Eleanora's loss broke her. Just like the rest of us, Shelagh had long awaited Eleanora's birth.

Next on our list was a flower shop to pick the vibrant colors that would surround Eleanora during the service. Something that would slightly ease the mood of the room and fill it with a fresh, uplifting scent.

We each got a bouquet for Eleanora. Written in gold letters on each bouquet was the relationship each person shared with Eleanora. There were two that read "granddaughter" and the one from us said "our little angel." In an effort to comfort me, my mother-in-law asked if she could buy me the bee slippers hanging on the wall. What I did not have the words to explain was that nothing would comfort me. She was desperately trying to buy my pain away, but it was a cost that could not be purchased with money. The pain and the ache in my heart were not something that would go away, but something I would have to learn to live with. Accepting that fact is just part of the process.

The next day, just like a couple expecting a baby, Nick and I went out shopping for an outfit for our sweet baby girl to wear. Only in our case, it was to be Eleanora's final one. Having followed the advice of a friend, we had not purchased newborn clothing, so we only had a few outfits in that size given as gifts in addition to some hand-me-downs from my cousin. Therefore, we had to go out and buy something that would fit her at only five days old. It was impossibly hard and I had to make several stops to cry. It was all so surreal.

We picked a one-piece outfit in white with purple dots and a big purple flower on the side. It suited her. She had a similar one in a larger size that I still have in my closet along with some other special outfits.

We next had to go to the funeral home to pick out a tiny urn, confirm the obituary I wrote was correct, and sign papers. From the get go, my Uncle Charlie had offered to pay for the service and any other charges that might arise along the way. He told me not to skimp on anything. I owe him so much, emotionally.

We walked through the aisles of urns and tried to find one that fit a baby. So many were too big, so many deemed not good enough, and so many did not capture how much she meant to us. When I saw one little, cherry wood box in which we could place a picture, I knew it was perfect. It reads:

Eleanora Lynn Scott
"Our little angel"
June 17-22, 2011

I gave the man from the funeral home the outfit we picked out, a white onesie, and even a newborn diaper as if she was getting ready for the day. I wanted her to be dressed like a baby and not a body. After all, she mattered (and still does) so much to me.

Chapter 8

A Life Lived

How do you sum up a life that has just begun? How can her life be measured simply in minutes, hours and days? As it turns out, Eleanora's life has continued to touch each day of mine as well as the lives of her siblings, but that was something I would only internalize much later. Early one morning, I was inspired to write Eleanora's obituary. Here it is just as the world saw it in the days after she passed.

Eleanora Lynn Scott, newborn daughter of Nicholas James Scott and Natalie Lynn Bishop Scott of Newark, DE, passed away on Wednesday, June 22, 2011.

Although Eleanora was here for only a short period of time, she brought so much joy to everyone who crossed her path. She truly was an angel of God on loan to us, her very proud parents. We will always remember you, Eleanora Lynn.

In addition to her parents, she is survived by her maternal grandmother, Lynn Betts, paternal grandmother, Tina Scott, and paternal grandfather, Ernest Scott, Jr. She was preceded in death by her pop-pop, Ken Betts.

A funeral service will be held at 7 pm on Tuesday, June 28, 2011, at the Spicer-Mullikin Funeral Home, 121 West Park Place, Newark, DE, where visitation will begin at 6 pm.

In lieu of flowers, contributions may be made to Easter Seals Delaware and Maryland's Eastern Shore, 61 Corporate Circle, New Castle, DE 19720.

Chapter 9

We Walk

The funeral service was scheduled, flowers were chosen, and the obituary was written. There was nothing left to do but wait. So, we walked. My mom said she would pick us up the next day to take us to Havre de Grace and walk. We walked away from it all for just a short time. Left the empty house still screaming of hardships to overcome and walked. Walked in the sunshine with no purpose. That was our band aid for the day. We ate soft shell crab sandwiches and to all the outside world we looked like a normal family enjoying a beautiful day. No one could see the gaping wounds we were just becoming accustomed to in those early days.

On Eleanora's fifth and sixth birthdays, we returned to Havre de Grace and walked this same path. On her sixth birthday, we released six balloons into the sky and watched them float above the trees into the clouds. We have followed this tradition for a couple of years now and tell our kids that we are sending them to Eleanora in heaven. They are excited to do this each year. They each got a turn to release balloons on her sixth birthday. As my oldest son released his pink flower balloon, he boldly exclaimed, "Happy birthday Eleanora!" There were onlookers ignorant as to what was going on, but that did not faze him one bit. Eleanora in heaven was his only focus as that is all he knows.

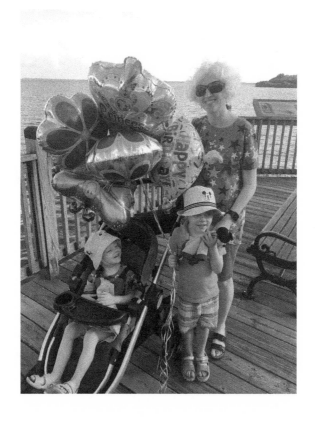

Chapter 10

It's Time...to Say Goodbye

I don't remember the day leading up to Eleanora's service. I remember waiting with both sadness and dread. Watching the hours pass. The day felt like it took forever. I knew this would be the last time I would ever see Eleanora on earth. I knew I wasn't allowed to pick her up, but that is all I wanted to do. Just sit in a rocker with her in my arms for the final time.

I wrote this entry in my journal the day of the service.

~~~

"Today is your funeral my little angel. Today is the last time I will ever get to touch your delicate skin, soft hair and chubby little cheeks. Someone else will dress your tiny little body in your last outfit. I am so sorry Mommy

isn't there to dress you. Soon you will be home again, but not in the same way. I will never be able to hold you again or comb my fingers through your pretty locks of hair. Daddy and I were so excited and looking forward to the future color of those golden locks.

Oh, Eleanora, everyone keeps telling me how strong I am, but how can I be strong with my heart in so many pieces? I love you so much and there is nothing I wouldn't give to have you back in my arms. We were supposed to spend the hot summer days together and instead I sit here without you, crying over my journal.

Daddy is taking down your things preparing for guests to come after the funeral. It is hard for me to watch because it means you are really gone and we are closing this chapter. Why was your chapter so short? You were supposed to close our books, lay us to rest."

***

Due to feeling overwhelmed by certain family members, I requested time for just me and Nick to see Eleanora. After us, close family members gathered around us and then the rest of her visitors.

While some people couldn't bear to look at Eleanora laying peacefully in her bassinet. Others were tender and gentle. My cousin Jen, who had not yet met Eleanora, said something along the lines of "now let's meet your baby girl." She treated me and my baby girl with respect and dignity. She treated me like a mom, even though my baby was no longer with us. It is these moments I hold dear.

After the service, Nick and I were the last to be in the room with Eleanora.

While Nick and I were saying goodbye, Hallelujah came on over the sound system. I explain later in this book that this is my song for Eleanora. Some lyrics are also included in a later chapter. This seemed to be the absolute best way to say goodbye. I leaned over and sang this song to her with tears streaming down my face. Though her life was short, I had learned the day after she was born that rubbing her chest calmed her down. I rubbed her chest, kissed her forehead, and told her Mommy would always love her. That is a promise that will never be broken.

Chapter 11

Now What?

A message from Pastor Leslie Cool for our daughter, Eleanora.

Eleanora Lynn Scott

Tuesday, June 28, 2011

In the name of the Father and of the Son and of the Holy Spirit.

Let us pray to the One who cares:

O Lord . . . This evening, we are not sure how to pray, except to throw ourselves upon your mercy. We grieve a loss that seems too big to endure. We grieve a loss that makes absolutely no sense to us. We need your help. Show us your love in the midst of our loss and pain.

Though this loss hurts, we do not ask that you numb our grief, but rather that you bind up our broken hearts. Help us to measure our grief in light of what we know about you, and so know and feel your gentle presence with us.

Lord, would you please comfort us in these moments as we seek assurance for life . . . life with hope and promise.

Heavenly Father, we know you understand pain and loss, for you watched your only Son die for our sins. In that moment, your heart was pierced. You KNOW what we feel. And so, we ask, save us from the pain of life and death, through Jesus Christ, Savior and Lord. Amen

Hear the Word of the Lord:

Lamentations 3:22-25 (NIV) . . . Because of the LORD's great love, we are not consumed, for his compassions never fail. 23 They are new every morning; great is your faithfulness. 24 I say to myself, "The LORD is my portion; therefore, I will wait for him." 25 The LORD is good to those whose hope is in him, to the one who seeks him;

The psalmist wrote:

Psalm 139:13-16 (NIV) . . . You created my inmost being; you knit me together in my mother's womb. 14 I praise you because I am fearfully and wonderfully made; your works are wonderful, I know that full well. 15 My frame was not hidden from you when I was made in the secret place. When I was woven together in the depths of the earth, 16 your eyes saw my unformed body. All the days ordained for me were written in your book before one of them came to be.

Psalm 46:1-3, 10 (NIV) . . . God is our refuge and strength, an ever-present help in trouble. 2 Therefore we will not fear, though the earth give way and the mountains fall into the heart of the sea, 3 though its waters roar and foam and the mountains quake with their surging.... And the Lord responded to the psalmist....10 "Be still, and know that I am God; I will be exalted among the nations, I will be exalted in the earth."

Jesus said:

John 14:1-3 (NLT). . . "Do not let your hearts be troubled. Trust in God; trust also in me. {2} In my Father's house are many rooms; if it were not so, I would have told you. I am going there to prepare a place for you. {3} And if I go and prepare a place for you, I will come back and take you to be with me that you also may be where I am."

John 14:27 (NIV). . . "Peace I leave with you; my peace I give you. I do not give to you as the world gives. Do not let your hearts be troubled and do not be afraid."

And the Apostle Paul wrote:

2 Corinthians 4:16-18 (NIV) . . . Therefore we do not lose heart. Though outwardly we are wasting away, yet inwardly we are being renewed day by day. 17 For our light and momentary troubles are achieving for us an eternal glory that far outweighs them all. 18 So we fix our eyes not on what is seen, but on what is unseen. For what is seen is temporary, but what is unseen is eternal.

This evening, we gather to measure and face our grief for the loss of a life not lived . . . Eleanora Lynn Scott, the newborn daughter of Nicholas James Scott and Natalie Lynn Bishop Scott, traded time for eternity on Wednesday, June 22, 2011. Eleanora was 5 days young. We grieve, not because we have known and lost Eleanora, but because we have lost Eleanora before we knew her . . . to fully love her.

And so . . . our grief is for a life not lived. We are left to grieve the loss of experiences that will not happen . . . late night feedings and the subsequent exhaustion; scrubbed knees, tears, mommy's hugs & kisses and colorful band aides; school, new math not understood, sports, scary boyfriends . . . and graduation; college, another graduation, the job search, wedding plans, the long-awaited grandchild.

It is in this kind of grief that we are tempted to become stuck on the hard questions . . . Why? Why me? I would like to suggest a healthier question . . . "Now what?" . . . a question directed heavenward.

Natalie and Nick . . . I have no answers to . . . Why? or Why me? But I want to remind you that the answers lie in the depth of God's endless grace and mercy and love. Oh, for sure, you may not feel this deep love . . . today, or tomorrow / next week. But you will . . . you will.

At first . . . I wanted to remind you of the story of David when his child became sick; of how he fasted and prayed, begging God to save his sick child. God did not. And after the child's death, David stood up and faced the rest of his life. This story is not quite for you . . . not tonight. But you will be like David; you'll get up and continue with your lives.

And I won't insult your intelligence or play with your hearts with promises you know, but may not be ready to embrace. God makes no mistakes. True, but hardly a comfort tonight. You will see Eleanora in heaven . . . someday. Also, true . . . you will . . . but you just want to hold her here and now.

In a panic over the weekend, as my computer screen remained empty for hours, I thought stories of Jesus and the little children might comfort you. Knowing that Eleanora was in Jesus' arms could bring comfort. I'm sure this will help . . . later.

My most successful attempt was a quick study of the life of Job . . . Job was a rich man . . . a man very content with life. Job walked apart from sin. And yet . . . God allowed Satan to mess with his life. Job lost his flocks and herds and servants. Job lost his children. Job lost everything that was measured as wealth. And then Job lost his good health. Job was left with . . . friends who accused him of hiding his sins, and a loving wife who said: "Get it over with. Curse God and die." (Job 2:9 NIV)

In all of this . . . Job did not sin. Sure, he questioned God's actions, or inaction. He wanted his day in court to prove he was in no way at fault. Eventually . . . God showed up, quickly set his so-called friends straight, and opened Job's eyes to see the wonders of God. Job was overwhelmed, and worshipped our great God.

In the end . . . God blessed Job . . . He restored his wealth, filled his house again with children. But I have few prophetic abilities. I do not know the status of your womb and heart, or what you might yet be able to bear. I cannot pretend to know how God might bless you in the future.

But I know that Job's story might be one that will feed you . . . later on. When you do, study closely the names of his three daughters . . . Jemimah – dovelike – or – like the sea; Keziah – fragrant spice; and Keren-Happuch – colorful eye makeup. Each name is a word embracing riotous excess. Job captured in names God's ability to over bless his children. Especially after a loss.

As I mentioned a few moments ago, any answers we might discover are hidden in the depths of God's mercy and grace and love. To know God . . . is to begin to know what he might be doing in our lives. Allow me to leave you with three truths about God . . . there are many, many more, but these three might touch you tonight.

Jeremiah 29:11 (NIV). . . "For I know the plans I have for you," declares the LORD, "plans to prosper you and not to harm you, plans to give you hope and a future."

Our nearsightedness does not allow us to view our life stories from the beginning to the end. And when we stand in the mess or loss of today, tomorrow fails to be attractive. But God has already been there . . . at the very end of each and every life story. So, when he says he is out for our very best, we can KNOW that he knows what he is talking about.

In time . . . your mind will overtake your emotions, you'll remember what you KNOW about our God . . . and he'll help you see what he needs you to know.

Psalm 61:1-3 (NIV) . . . Hear my cry, O God; listen to my prayer. 2 From the ends of the earth I call to you, I call as my heart grows faint; lead me to the rock that is higher than I. 3 For you have been my refuge, a strong tower against the foe.

In these hard days . . . days of grieving, you'll want to be alone. You'll want to retreat into a safe place, away from well-meaning but often less than helpful people. That's okay; that's not a bad thing. Protect yourselves! But allow me to remind you that God is not just a person . . . like you and me. God is a safe place. ALWAYS! The psalmist knew God as a rock, a fortress, a strong tower, a very safe place. In your grief . . . remember God . . . your best safe place.

Romans 8:26 (NIV) . . . In the same way, the Spirit helps us in our weakness. We do not know what we ought to pray for, but the Spirit himself intercedes for us with groans that words cannot express.

Herein is a promise that we can hardly grasp. God longs to finish our unspoken prayers. What I see best in these words is that when my prayers run dry . . . no words to express myself, no words to say to or at

God, he steps in and finishes my prayers. Keep talking with God, even if you end up sobbing in his arms. He'll carry you along.

You see . . . Natalie and Nick, it's not so much a search for the answers to "Why?" or "Why me?" as it is knowing the One who knows. Through your tears . . . and there will be many; through your tears, gaze toward God . . . expectantly. Your hope is not in understanding the "Why?" of what has already happened. Your hope is in understanding "Now what?" as you join hands and hearts and step forward into what might be. God will answer this question!

Let us pray:

Heavenly Father . . . author of life and death, we trust You to bind our broken hearts, and to mend . . . our torn lives.

We pray for Your Spirit to move in our hearts and lives, ever and always drawing us unto Yourself and the life You have promised.

Strengthen us to live the kind of lives that glorify You and point others to the Jesus Eleanora now fully knows.

Hold us tight, our Father, as we press on with your promises and Your truth ever before us. Amen.

Part 2

The Sun Will Rise

Chapter 12

The Clouds Will Part

He gives power to the weak and strength to the powerless. Even youths will become weak and tired and young men will fall in exhaustion. But those who trust in the Lord will find new strength. They will soar high on wings like eagles. They will run and not grow weary. They will walk and not faint.

Isaiah 40:29-31 (NLT)

I wish this was a story of quick healing and immediately finding inner peace. I wish I could tell you a tale of finding God's purpose right after Eleanora's death. But this is not that tale. Mine is a tale that took years.

It is a tale of love, hate, grace, fear, disappointment, and an unending devotion from a God who is a perfect Father. Even though we all must walk our own course along this journey, I hope your road to healing is much faster and much less painful than mine. Despite the length of time it took for me to find peace and make my way back to God, I think it was all meant to be. At the end of that painful path, which is in reality endless, I have a deep and meaningful relationship with God that I never would've known if things had not gotten ugly. He still loves me, cares for me, and knows the depths of my heart. And better yet, I know His too. I have a deeper glimpse into who my Father truly is all because of his faithfulness to me.

Chapter 13

Ship Wreck

As the months wore on after Eleanora's death, I found comfort in unexpected places. Dancing around with our dog, Tater, to the song "Moves Like Jagger" by Maroon 5 was the first time I remember smiling, even laughing. A promise that life could and would go on. At first, I felt guilty for laughing about something so silly, but then I felt that Eleanora would not want me to be miserable. So, we danced and I laughed. To this day, every time that song comes on, I sing out loud and smile about the first time I laughed thanks to the lyrics, "I've got the moves like Tater. I've got the moves like Panda (our other dog). I've got the mooooooves like Jagger." And it is okay to laugh even if it still hurts.

I also found the advice below on a forum. Someone had recently lost their friend and was heartbroken. Here is one person's reply:

"Alright, here goes. I'm old. What that means is that I've survived (so far) and a lot of people I've known and loved did not. I've lost friends, best friends, acquaintances, co-workers, grandparents, mom, relatives, teachers, mentors, students, neighbors, and a host of other folks. I have no children, and I can't imagine the pain it must be to lose a child. But here's my two cents.

I wish I could say you get used to people dying. I never did. I don't want to. It tears a hole through me whenever somebody I love dies, no matter the circumstances. But I don't want it to "not matter." I don't want it to be something that just passes. My scars are a testament to the love and the relationship that I had for and with that person. And if the scar is deep, so was the love. So be it. Scars are a testament to life. Scars are a testament that I can love deeply and live deeply and be cut, or even gouged, and that I can heal and continue to live and continue to love. And the scar tissue is stronger than the original flesh ever was. Scars are a testament to life. Scars are only ugly to people who can't see.

As for grief, you'll find it comes in waves. When the ship is first wrecked, you're drowning, with wreckage all around you. Everything floating around you reminds you of the beauty and the magnificence of the ship that was, and is no more. And all you can do is float. You find some piece of the wreckage and you hang on for a while. Maybe it's some physical thing. Maybe it's a happy memory or a photograph. Maybe it's a person who is also floating. For a while, all you can do is float. Stay alive.

In the beginning, the waves are 100 feet tall and crash over you without mercy. They come 10 seconds apart and don't even give you time to catch your breath. All you can do is hang on and float. After a while, maybe weeks, maybe months, you'll find the waves are still 100 feet tall, but they come further apart. When they come, they still crash all over you and wipe you out. But in between, you can breathe, you can function. You never know what's going to trigger the grief. It might be a song, a picture, a street intersection, the smell of a cup of coffee. It can be just about anything...and the wave comes crashing. But in between waves, there is life.

Somewhere down the line, and it's different for everybody, you find that the waves are only 80 feet tall. Or 50 feet tall. And while they still come, they come further apart. You can see them coming. An anniversary, a birthday, or Christmas, or landing at O'Hare. You can see it coming, for the most part, and prepare yourself. And when it washes over you, you know that somehow you will, again, come out the other side. Soaking wet, sputtering, still hanging on to some tiny piece of the wreckage, but you'll come out.

Take it from an old guy. The waves never stop coming, and somehow you don't really want them to. But you learn that you'll survive them. And other waves will come. And you'll survive them too. If you're lucky, you'll have lots of scars from lots of loves. And lots of shipwrecks."

Shared with permission from G. Snow

Chapter 14

Trust

I think with a new loss, the words of the song "Trust In You" will sting, but they will also resonate with you. I spent many days crying out for answers asking God to move mountains and part waters. It wasn't until I trusted in Him and in His plan that I felt peace. I still question God sometimes, but in my heart, I know He has a plan.

"Trust in You"

When You don't move the mountains
I'm needing You to move
When You don't part the waters
I wish I could walk through

When You don't give the answers
As I cry out to You
I will trust, I will trust, I will trust in You

My pastor recently gave a sermon that was titled "Make Friends with the Fish." In the sermon he discussed the story of Jonah and the whale. Jonah spent three days in the whale and as terrible as that situation was, it was better than the alternative. God used that whale to protect Jonah and used that time to teach him. When it was God's time, Jonah was spit out on the beach safely. The three days in the whale were compared to a time of struggle, like the loss of your baby, and in God's time you will come out on the other side unharmed, protected by an amazing Father who loves you. A Father who is with you the entire time you are in the belly of the whale. For me, as I mentioned before, I felt God's arms around my family as I held Eleanora in the emergency room. I felt Him grieving with me. I can picture it in my mind. He walked hand in hand with us through every step of grief and continues to do so, still holding me whenever I cry. He is with you too.

I don't know what your out-of-the-whale moment will be. On the other hand, I have been in the belly of the whale just like you. I have felt the hopelessness, the desire to see the light again, the depression, jealousy, anguish, and loneliness. I have been there. I can promise you there is life on the other side. You may stink of fish – wearing the scars of your pain. You may not be the same person. However, you will survive. You will see light again.

⁓

"Trust in You"

(Lauren Daigle/Michael Farren/Paul Mabury)

Letting go of every single dream
I lay each one down at Your feet

Every moment of my wandering
Never changes what You see
I try to win this war
I confess, my hands are weary, I need Your rest
Mighty warrior, king of the fight
No matter what I face You're by my side
When You don't move the mountains
I'm needing You to move
When You don't part the waters
I wish I could walk through
When You don't give the answers
As I cry out to You
I will trust, I will trust, I will trust in You
Truth is, You know what tomorrow brings
There's not a day ahead You have not seen
So let all things be my life and breath
I want what You want Lord and nothing less
When You don't move the mountains
I'm needing You to move
When You don't part the waters
I wish I could walk through
When You don't give the answers
As I cry out to You
I will trust, I will trust, I will trust in You
I will trust in You
You are my strength and comfort
You are my steady hand
You are my firm foundation
The rock on which I stand
Your ways are always higher
Your plans are always good
There's not a place where I'll go
You've not already stood
When You don't move the mountains
I'm needing You to move

When You don't part the waters
I wish I could walk through
When You don't give the answers
As I cry out to You
I will trust, I will trust, I will trust in You
I will trust in You
I will trust in You
I will trust in You

Chapter 15

Meaning in the Mess

Lord, remember my suffering and how I have no home. Remember the misery and suffering. I remember them well. And I am very sad. But I have hope when I think of this: The Lord's love never ends. His mercies never stop. They are new every morning. Lord, your loyalty is great. I say to myself, "The Lord is what I have left. So I have hope." The Lord is good to those who put their hope in him. He is good to those who look to him for help. It is good to wait quietly for the Lord to save.

Lamentations 3:19-26 (ICB)

Sometimes, the hurt feels so new, so painful, that it seems too much for one person to bear. Now as we inch painfully towards Eleanora's sixth birthday, one we will not celebrate with her here, the memories feel so distant, so fuzzy, so unimaginably unreal.

I lived so long with hate and anger. I wasted so many years yearning for what I lost, for what everyone else around me had. I found this journal entry from 2015 and, with the idea of being vulnerable, I share it with you. Talking with friends has shown me this is just how I viewed myself. I am way too harsh a critic. Just because I was upset or angry does not mean I did not find joy at all. There was plenty of joy and happiness. There was also envy and fear.

"The day I said goodbye was the day it all began. Funny how a story begins with a goodbye. I changed that day. I started down a rode of a whirlwind of emotions, but in the end held onto pure jealousy. I became someone I did not like. People kept telling me what a wonderful person and mother I was, but they did not know. They didn't know the awful thoughts I had about my life, my husband, the world I lived in and myself. I became someone I did not like. It wasn't Eleanora's fault, but that is where the hate started to spiral out of control spewing its hideous shadow over everything in my life.

I was desperate to come up for air and change, but the blackness was so gripping and so intertwined with everything in my life. I felt there was no escape. I had lived this way for so long and although I did not like myself or living that way I had no idea where to begin. One day after overreacting to my oldest son and feeling the "mom guilt" from my actions, I started to write. It felt good to get it all out on paper. There it was in front of me in black and white. I am someone I do not like and I need to make a change."

I lived so long with God begging to come in and me pushing Him out and locking the door in His face. I was still going to church and still believed there was a God, but would not let Him too close to me. He waited for me. He knocked gently and when I was ready, I let Him back in. I released my hurt to Him. God says in Matthew 11:28-30 (NIV) "Come to me, all you who are weary and burdened, and I will give you rest. Take my yoke upon you and learn from me, for I am gentle and humble in heart, and you will find rest for your souls. For my yoke is easy and my burden is light."

Ever since I let go of the tight hold I had on my loss, I have felt a love, peace and meaning in the mess. I don't mean I understand why Eleanora was taken, but rather I know with assured faith that there is a reason. Her life was not a mistake. My loss of her was not a mistake. God mourned with me. God sees the whole picture as my pastor, Les, said in his sermon for her. He knows our life from beginning to end, long or short.

When I looked back at my journal entries from right after Eleanora passed, I found an entry on July 12 that offers so much peace. I wish I would have held onto this so I did not waste so much time. I hope it offers you the same amount of peace it did for me. This shows how the tides of grieve come and go. One day is clear and peaceful and the next can be full of anger, self-loathing or torrents of tears. Let those emotions come but also let them go. Anger is not a lifeline. The sea will calm again and the blue skies will return. It is a journey to say the least.

~~~~~

"At times, I feel clarity and at peace because I believe in God and know you are with Him.

I am no longer angry with God. As Les (my pastor) says, He makes no mistakes. That means, Eleanora, as much as it kills me, you were only meant to be here for five days. You should know the ten months in my womb and those five days were the happiest I have ever known. Even though I was robbed of you, at least I had you to begin with. Just the two of us shared so many secret moments when you were growing in my womb. I am so very grateful for all those kicks and wiggles. Although five days is way too short. I had five days. Some moms do not even get that. For me, those days were pure ecstasy. You filled my days with joy and my nights with secret moments for just us to share.

I cannot promise that tomorrow I will be at peace and write this clearly, but today or in this moment, Eleanora, God is giving me peace. I am so grateful to know Him. One day I will know God like you know Him. He will gather me in his arms and hold and protect me too."

I hope with time you find a meaning in your mess and embrace the peace that God has to offer you.

Chapter 16

My Heart Goes Out to You, Mom I Never Met

"Be kind, for everyone you meet is fighting a hard battle."

— *Ian MacLaren*

During one of my routine ultrasounds, the tech said something about fluid in Eleanora's kidneys. She told us it was nothing to worry about and moved on. We looked questioningly at each other, but brushed it off since it was supposedly nothing to worry about.

When my OB read the ultrasound notes, she was outraged. She sent us straight to the hospital to have another ultrasound to be absolutely sure Eleanora was safe. While we were waiting in the curtained off rooms, we overheard a conversation with the patient next to us. Our conversation stopped in its tracks as we heard the doctor explain to the mom that her baby had a heart defect. My heart broke for that poor mom. There I was having something rechecked that turned out to be nothing more than Eleanora needing to pee really badly and this poor woman's life was falling to pieces around her. I wanted to jump up and go give her a hug and tell her it would be okay. I didn't, of course, since I was not supposed to have heard the news. I have no idea what happened to that mom or to her baby. I don't know if the baby lived or not.

I tell this story because I often think of that mom. I felt so bad for her not knowing if the heart defect was something they could fix and then four months later I was burying my own perfectly healthy baby. Nothing could have prepared us for what happened to our baby girl.

Chapter 17

Immeasurable Purpose

You saw my body as it was formed. All the days planned for me were
written in your book before I was one day old.

Psalm 139:16 (ICB)

God has a purpose for Eleanora. Her life was short and to some people
insignificant, but, to God, her life is measured in more than days,
weeks or years. Her life is measured in so much more. Eleanora's life
and impact on our family is endless. Her story has sent ripples around
the world. She has touched people in ways we cannot understand. Even

those that never met her felt her loss. She has a purpose and she is still fulfilling it even from heaven.

I know this to be true about Eleanora and your baby too. Your baby matters and so does your story. Don't stop telling your story. It may make people feel uncomfortable, but you have no idea the impact it may have on someone else's life.

Recently, I had a friend share with me her experience of losing her child. She felt ashamed and never shared her story with anyone except her husband. She opened up to me because she knew I could understand her loss. She held onto that secret for decades, but my story touched her so much that she felt ready to set that secret free. Once her story was out, she felt peace and acceptance. It was my honor to share that with her and offer her the words of comfort she needed to heal.

Don't be ashamed of your story. Don't be ashamed of your feelings. Find someone with whom you can trust and release your story. Don't keep it trapped inside. Give it wings and let it fly. You have no clue who it will touch and how far it will go.

I felt guilty for a long time after Eleanora died. I think that is why it took so much longer to heal. I looked back and blamed myself for her death. Her death made me second guess my instincts.

I was talking with a friend about how my brain could not let go of June 22 and everything I should have done. I told her every detail of that morning. This friend is the type that does not "sugar coat" her words. I braced myself for judgement. I knew she was going to confirm everything I feared. However, I was met with the opposite response. She asked how I could possibly think that Eleanora's death was my fault. She told me I was being completely irrational and I needed to let it go. She was not saying it to appease me, she was saying it as a matter of fact. She was the key that unlocked the chains I had grown to know so well. My life was different after that day. Every time I start to slip down that slope of blaming myself again, her words ring in my ears.

A couple of days after Eleanora died, some friends dropped off a bag of food at the door. They texted me to let me know they were thinking of me and the food was at the door. It was such a kind and gentle gesture. Neither of them was a mom yet, so the gesture meant that much more to me.

About a month later they came back with another friend and let me share my story of her birth. Very few people got to hear the story. It was so quickly overshadowed by her death and people trying to forget she existed, for their comfort or as not to upset me. However, as you probably know that makes things so much worse.

My friends let me share my birth story as if Eleanora was sleeping quietly upstairs in her basinet. They let me feel like a "normal" mom. We ate and laughed. For a little bit of time, it felt like everything was okay. This time of being able to speak her name without people cringing or shying away meant the world to me. I am so grateful for these ladies and I do not think they will ever understand the impact they had on my life during that impossibly difficult time. They recognized me as the mom I was.

Around that time, I wrote this journal entry.

"My precious child, today is very hard. Daddy went back to work today and I am alone in the house for the first time since we lost you. Today should have been a happy day. I was so excited for your first fourth of July. Grammy bought you an outfit and hair bows that would have looked great on you. You would have been the biggest, brightest firework in our lives. But instead, I am here alone with a gaping hole in my heart and life. All of your stuff is packed up in your room. Eleanora, life is empty, hurtful and hard without you. I am still looking and begging God for the meaning in all of this and coming up short.

Eleanora, you are home with us again. I made a special place with your blanket and candle. You'll always be my baby and I will never forget you.

I go back to work tomorrow and I am scared. I know it is too soon, but I can't sit around the house without you to take care of while everyone else is at work. We had a lot of days alone while you were growing in my belly. I was so happy then, watching you grow, move, kick, wiggle and hiccup. I felt like I had a purpose as a Mommy. Now I feel empty. My soul feels drained and I am emotionally tired.

I was so blessed to have you, Eleanora. You showed me what living really is. It is growing a baby and stopping everything for her. Seeing who your real friends are. Watching your relationship with your husband grow stronger and unbreakable. It is loving someone so much that you change everything for them. Being proud of stretch marks and a chubby belly because it shows you are a mom. Thank you, Eleanora, for showing me all that. I love you so much and always will. I bet you are the most beautiful angel in heaven. I love you!"

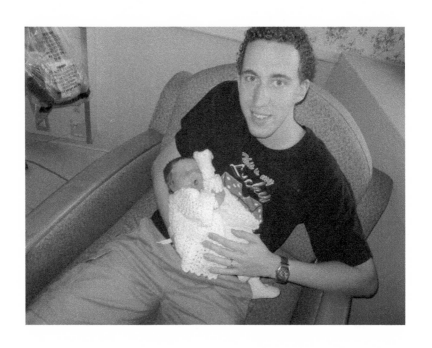

Chapter 18

You Are A Mother

About a month after losing Eleanora I found the poem, **"What Makes a Mother" by Jennifer Wasik**. It brought so much comfort to me. The first few times I read it, I cried. Imagining God and Eleanora speaking the words in the poem directly to me always brings tears to my eyes. Thinking of her whispering these words in my ear brings so much joy and comfort.

I miss my Mommy oh so much
But I visit her each day.
I stroke her hair and kiss her check
And whisper in her ear
"Mommy don't be sad today,
I'm your baby and I'm here."

The above content is just part of the beautiful poem by Jennifer Wasik written in memory of her son Zachery. I encourage you to find the entire poem at: https://www.irisremembers.com/poemsandstories/viewPoem.cfm?poemID=200

I think it is so important that you remember you are a mom, forever. No one can take that away from you. People may trivialize the idea of that and tell you different things, but that baby is always your baby and you are always their mommy.

I always tell people I have three children. Just because Eleanora is in heaven, does not mean she is no longer my child. I will always be her Mommy no matter the distance or the situation.

Chapter 19

Always Your Mommy

I wrote this poem on November 13, 2011

I Will Always Be Your Mommy

Natalie Scott
Written for Eleanora Lynn with love

I will always be your Mommy,
Though you're no longer here.
No longer can I hear your cries
Or wipe away your tears.

I will always be your Mommy.
In my heart you'll forever be.
Your soft skin, your sweet smell,
Once here is now a distant memory.

You'll always be my baby,
Though you're no longer in my arms.
The house is filled with your spirit
And my heart left with scars.

You'll always be my baby.
Not a single day goes by,
That you're not on my mind
And I'm not asking why?

Remember baby, I'll always be your Mommy
And though it seems we are far apart
You'll always be my baby
And you'll always be with me in my heart.

Chapter 20

My Five Stages of Grief

My friend Tamar has written two books about the loss of her baby. ("Letting Go of Baby" and "What's Next?: A guide to dealing with grief after a loss.") In her second book, she explores the stages of grief. She asked me to write what those five stages looked like for me after losing a newborn baby. These are the entries that appear in her book.

The First stage of grief is Denial/Isolation

Entailed in this stage is one's struggle with acknowledging and or dealing with reality. During this stage, the mother or father may immediately deny the fact that they really lost their child when they first receive the news. This is a normal response and is actually the way the mind defends itself from being tremendously affected by a traumatic experience. Losing a baby can cause a mom or parent to feel numb. A mom or dad may not cry or sometimes even speak about what happened for days, weeks or, on some occasions, months. They feel empty, they continue to avoid social relationships, and their loss increases (Comer, 2001).

It is hard to deny the fact that she was gone when her absence was present everywhere we looked. Her room was filled with all of her clothes waiting to be worn, toys to be played with and other things that go along with a baby. Her bassinet where she laid her beautiful head just the night before was now painfully and deafeningly empty. It was hard to deny that she was gone when her cooing no longer woke me up at night to nurse. The heaviness of my empty arms reminded me that she was no longer here.

However, when they were doing CPR to bring her back to us I kept asking if she would be okay. Surely, they could bring her back, I thought against all reason. I was just holding a happy, healthy baby one minute and what felt like the next minute doctors were fighting for her next breath. It all happened in an instant.

While we were in the emergency room watching the group of doctors and nurses work to save her I prayed over and over to please let her live. Begging God not to take her away from us. I pleaded with God for a miracle. Leaving my precious, baby girl alone in the hospital emergency room was one of the hardest things I have ever had to do. It was hard to deny that she was gone at that point.

The second stage of grief is Anger

During this phase a mother, father or sibling may become irritable, short in conversation, and or verbally or physically aggressive. They might look at the persons around them and feel envy, jealousy, and rage over their health and vigor (Vander Zanden, 2003). Some individuals are angry with the unborn child. We may resent the person for causing us pain or for leaving us (Axelrod, 2006)

I was never angry with Eleanora. In my mind, she did not want to leave. I have gone through several stages of anger. I go in and out of this stage still, five years later. At the beginning, I was angry at every mother who had a baby after Eleanora passed away and got to keep their baby. I was, and still am, jealous of every first-time mom, which is what I was, who naively has and keeps their baby. Since I lost a girl and then later had two boys, this stage of anger/jealousy is a constant ebb and flow in my life as I watch other little girls grow up. I will never know what my little girl would be like. That thought slips me in to the stage of depression.

The third stage of grief is Bargaining

In this phase, individuals are trying to regain control over their lives. It's a vain expression of hope that the bad news is reversible. Secretly, we may make a deal with God or our higher power in an attempt to postpone the inevitable (Axelrod, 2006). Parents may start to question themselves and the decisions that they made prior to losing their baby. Statements and/or thoughts may start off with "If I only had . . ., they should have . . ., I should have known . . .". In this stage, one may be fixated on what happened and may find themselves constantly searching for answers regarding the loss of the baby. While this is a normal response, staying in this stage may prevent someone from living a fulfilled life.

I spent many sleepless nights for years focused on what, in my mind, I did wrong. If I would have done this... I should have done that... I go over every detail of the morning she passed away. I beat myself mentally. In moments of clarity I know there was nothing more that could have been done, but when I am trapped in the clutches of these evil thoughts I cannot see passed my perceived faults. My way of tamping down these negative thoughts were to constantly have noise, music or television, to distract my mind from reliving the same painful moments over and over. Family, friends, even doctors and one close friend who said just the right words, assured me there was nothing more that could have been done and I am more confident that I did everything I could have done. Now, I only occasionally find myself questioning the events of that day.

The fourth stage of grief is Depression

Anger can often be a sign that someone is depressed. Sadness and regret predominate this type of depression. It is our quiet preparation to separate and to bid our loved one farewell (Axelrod, 2006). A parent may feel like they have lost motivation and possess no desire to continue on with daily activities during the stage of depression, or may lose the desire to spend time with their friends especially those that have children or somehow remind them of their baby. During this stage, one may also blame themselves or others for what happened. A parent may also continue to replay words or specific scenarios surrounding the incident which can contribute to the cycle of depression.

Anger/jealousy, bargaining/questioning myself and depression were my constant companions. While I no longer had my baby to hold I was encircled with these constant emotions sending me up and down a roller coaster for years. I believe the grieving process can take a lifetime until we are reunited with our babies in heaven. I continue to slip in and out of this stage as I watch little girls grow up. It was hard for me to even watch my second child achieve milestones my daughter never had a chance to achieve. At the beginning, I avoided any pregnant mother, baby showers, baby stores and anything to do with babies. I didn't go to celebrations at work as a way to avoid a pregnant coworker. To me, it felt like their swelling bellies were mocking me. I closed my office door and avoided happy chatter about the upcoming baby and subsequent delivery. No one understood my misery. It was a very lonely and isolating time for me.

The fifth stage of grief is Acceptance

In the acceptance stage, they no longer struggle against death (in this case that of their child) but make peace with it, (Vander Zanden, 2003). It is during this phase that a parent recognizes that they have to continue on and adjust their minds and lives to change from what they were expecting. When someone has begun to accept their loss, this does not mean that they are fine with losing their child, but they realize they will have to continue on without the physical being of their child.

I am not sure when I reached this stage, but for me, acceptance meant celebrating her life. We celebrate her birthday every year and find other ways to remember her and keep her memory alive. We talk about her with our other kids. We talk about how she is still with us in our hearts and guiding us. When people ask how many kids I have I include her. Although I have accepted she is not here on earth, talking about and including her helps me. Acceptance, for me, is every day. Every day I have to acknowledge that I have to go on without her. I carry her memories in my heart so I know she is never far away.

Chapter 21

What I Have Learned

"Let me tell you something you already know. The world ain't all sunshine and rainbows. It's a very mean and nasty place, and I don't care how tough you are, it will beat you to your knees and keep you there permanently if you let it. You, me, or nobody is gonna hit as hard as life. But it ain't about how hard you hit. It's about how hard you can get hit and keep moving forward; how much you can take and keep moving forward."

— *Rocky Barboa*

I have learned that I am strong. If you are reading this book, then you are too. You have survived or are surviving something that it seems you shouldn't have. You are strong in spirit, an emotional rock, even though you don't feel that way, especially if your loss was recent. You are strong physically too. You are living and breathing even though it feels like there is an unimaginable weight on your chest that threatens to squeeze the life out of you. You are surviving against all odds. You are seeking help or the comfort found in these pages. You are living and you are strong.

I survived the death of my daughter. I survived people's thoughtless comments and actions. I have survived the feeling of loneliness in a world not meant for a grieving mom. I walk with my head held high. I talk about Eleanora like anyone would speak of their child. She is still my daughter and always will be. I won't be silenced and neither should you.

I have learned that people can be cruel. Their words and actions can be like salt in your already gaping wound. Even when the wound feels like it is healing or has healed, those words or actions can rip it open again and fill you with an incredible amount of pain. During Eleanora's funeral arrangements, someone thought it was appropriate to pull out their phone, read a text message, and then show everyone at the table the picture of a lawn mower attached in the text. The whole table, including the man from the funeral home, was stunned into silence. I look back and imagine all the things I wish I had said, but at the time I was an empty version of myself. I had nothing to give or say.

I have learned that mentioning Eleanora can quiet a room in a split second. It makes people run from me or avoid me as if her death were contagious. I can't change how they feel, but their discomfort will not keep me from talking about her.

I have also learned that people can be incredibly kind with words expressed through all mediums. I have learned that Eleanora is not just on my mind or that of my husband's, but on the minds of people who never knew her. I don't carry the burden alone.

I have learned that people look up to me because I kept going after she took her last breath. Where I saw weakness, others saw strength.

What I see as failure, others see as success. In fact, during our 2017 fundraiser for March of Dimes, a friend posted this on her Facebook page to help raise funds:

> **Elise Brogan** – "I get to meet a lot of really awesome people #becauseoflularoe. Some of them change my life forever. The Scott family are some of those people. Fun and spunky with 2 typically crazy toddler boys, you would think they are your average family if you saw them at the mall or the playground.
>
> But as soon as you talk to Natalie or Nicholas you'll find out that there is a little girl that, though she's no longer here on earth, is vibrantly alive in their family. Nick and Natalie lost their first child, Eleanora, when she was just 5 days old.
>
> But they never really lost her. They have kept her alive in everything they do. Talking about Eleanora is not a delicate topic at the Scott house, it's encouraged.
>
> Most of us cannot fathom what we would do or say or how we would carry on if we lost a child. I pray that I never find out, but I like to think that I'd be like Natalie. And in fact, some of the panic that overcomes me any time I think about the possibility of something happening to Finn or Betsy is soothed a way when I think about the Scott family."

I had no idea she felt this way about me until I saw her beautiful words on social media. I learned that I am an example of what to do. I always felt like I was the prime example of what not to do.

I learned that people will surprise you in so many bad ways, but also in so many wonderful ways! Some of the hurt people caused after we lost Eleanora is unfathomable, but over the last several years we have had so much kindness from others.

I have learned that I don't need to get over it. I'll never get over it. I will always carry this loss and the emotions that come with it. I think that is okay. I can move forward with my loss, but never get over it. Forward motion is good. At first, sitting still is good. Letting the waves of emotion lap over you is good, but one day you'll stand up out of the tide and walk forward carrying the weight with you. Don't get over it, but don't get stuck drowning in the ocean. When you are ready, stand up. You'll look different and many people may not see the difference, but you won't be the you that you were yesterday. You are forever changed.

I have learned that I can't do it alone. I have learned to trust God with my feelings and sorrow and know He will be there for me and with me. We are not meant to do it alone. Believe me, I tried and I spent those years in the darkness. I saw the light only when I finally took His outstretched hand.

I have learned and continue to learn how Eleanora's loss impacts the lives of her siblings who never met her. They are growing up to be that much more interesting and special having their sister in heaven and knowing she is still very much a part of their lives. They have another level of empathy that others don't have. We talk about her openly in our house. Pierce tells me how much he misses her even though he never knew her here on earth. They know her in their own special way.

I have learned that kids, not just my own, understand loss better than adults do. Kids have said the sweetest things to me. Right after I lost Eleanora, I was babysitting kids I know well. Their mom told them what happened. She also lost a child and so understands the feeling of loss. We were eating dinner and the little girl noticed the necklace I was wearing depicting a mom and baby intertwined. She looked at me and said, "Your baby is beautiful!" I know she meant my necklace, but part of me thinks she could see Eleanora too.

My son, Pierce, has said so many wonderful things concerning his sister. He is wise beyond his years in this respect. One day, I was crying because I missed Eleanora. He asked me why I was crying. When I told him I just missed Eleanora, he said, "Mommy you don't need to miss her. She lives in your heart." I had to hold back even more tears to respond, "Yes, she does Pierce. Yes, she does."

You'll learn these lessons and more along your journey. Yours won't be exactly the same, but you'll meet cruel, thoughtless people. Their words or actions will tear at your soul. I hope, for you, that you'll meet many more kind people that bring joy to your life and healing to your soul.

Chapter 22

Hallelujah

As I prefaced in a previous chapter, Hallelujah is my song for Eleanora. I include some of the lyrics to this song because I sang it to her over and over while I rocked my growing belly. When I hear it, I know she is with me. When I sing it, I feel her swaying along with the rhythm.

Leonard Cohen sings a slightly different version than that of Jeff Buckley or Pentatonix (one of my favorite bands. Their version is like heaven in a song). He finishes the song with these lines that I feel sum up our story.

"Hallelujah!"

And even though it all went wrong
I'll stand before the lord of song
With nothing on my tongue but hallelujah
Hallelujah, Hallelujah, Hallelujah, Hallelujah

"Hallelujah"

Jeff Buckley

Well, I heard there was a secret chord
That David played and it pleased the Lord
But you don't really care for music, do you?
Well it goes like this:
The fourth, the fifth, the minor fall and the major lift
The baffled king composing Hallelujah

Hallelujah, Hallelujah, Hallelujah, Hallelujah

Chapter 23

Endless Night

As you can see, I find comfort or solace in many places. The lyrics from the song "Endless Night" from The Lion King on Broadway are very personal to me. I can see my story in this song. Not just from losing my stepdad, but from losing Eleanora. She never promised me she wouldn't leave like the lyrics "you promised you'd be there," but it is an unsaid promise that a child will not die before a parent. And now we walk this path that is not familiar to most.

The song begins in the depths of despair, which you are probably feeling right now. It may feel like "Home is an empty dream lost to the night" and you feel alone in the darkness that surrounds you. In these moments, it is hard to imagine you will ever have a breakthrough. It feels like you are drowning in the sea of sorrow with no way out.

I can relate so well to the words in the song of holding on, grasping at straws, waiting to hear her cry or her voice one last time. I have begged just to hear one word or just to have one last hug. As it says in the song "one word, just a word will do to end this nightmare."

The song continues asking "when will the dawning break?" You may be asking. when will I feel okay again? For each person it is different. There is no method to it. And you may feel okay for awhile and then an anniversary comes along and breaks you again. Over time, you will find healing.

This song also offers a promise. The night will end, the clouds will clear and the sun will rise! Breathe my friends, the sun will rise. Hold onto that hope in your darkest hours and, there will be dark hours and days. Soon you will find the light and the sun will shine.

You may have never heard your baby's voice to begin with or ever again in the same way you had previously, but soon you'll learn to "hear" your child's voice within your heart. One day, you will meet your baby and hear your baby's voice, either for the first time, or once again.

This is how "Endless Night" ends.

I know that the night must end
I know that the sun will rise
And I'll hear your voice deep inside

Until we meet again, your voice will beat with the rhythm of my heart sweet child.

Chapter 24

Do What Is Right for You!

Giving up is easy. Just laying down and throwing in the towel, anyone can do that. But standing up and continuing to live and breathe when the world expects you to fall apart. That shows dignity. That deserves respect. And that is the example of true strength. You are that person!

As you already know, Eleanora's name is not a secret in our house. We tell people about her; her picture is hanging in our foyer with our other children and we talk about her openly with our kids. She is always included in our family because she is forever our daughter and their sister.

However, this isn't always easy for others to accept. At times it brings silence and an uncomfortable atmosphere. I have gotten used to this, but in your home, you have to choose what is right for you. Can you handle the rejection, silence, and exclusion? For me, it was worse to exclude Eleanora than to deal with how others felt. Everyone is different. Don't let anyone tell you how to handle your grief or how to approach this decision.

There are other unforeseen repercussions to the decision we made to always include Eleanora in our family and in our conversations with our children.

My children hurt for Eleanora. They long to meet the sister they never had a chance to meet. My older son often says he misses her and wishes she would come back. He is not repeating my words. These are straight from the heart of a child who wishes he could know his sister on earth. He has even prayed at night that God will send Eleanora back to earth so he can play with her.

Eleanora and Pierce have a special connection that I cannot begin to understand, but I know he wishes she was more tangible. He told me about a dream he recently had that she sent a balloon down from heaven to pick him up. At first, he was afraid because I could not reach him, but when he got to heaven there was Eleanora. He told me she was wearing a pink dress. She had blonde hair and blue eyes "just like we do." She told him all about God and how wonderful He is. When they were done talking and playing, she sent him back to earth floating on her balloon, which he later sent back up to her.

I believe this was a gift from Eleanora to ease the pain her brother is feeling. In my heart, though it seems impossible, I believe every word Pierce said. Children have amazing connections that I don't think we could ever hope to understand. As I've said before, Eleanora will not stop touching our lives. Her five days on earth cannot begin to measure her true impact on our lives and those we know.

Chapter 25

A Moment of Clarity

You intended to harm me, but God intended it all for good. He brought me to this position so I could save the lives of many people.

Genesis 50:20 (NLT)

I wrote the following at some point shortly after Eleanora died. I found it in the box with everything from her service, including the sympathy cards that came pouring in from all directions filling our house with reminders we were not alone, the pink bows from her flower arrangements, and the sign in book with the teddy bear on the cover.

I had long forgotten the sense of purpose I had found in those early days. Here is what I wrote:

"A Moment of clarity"

God makes no mistakes. We were selected for a reason. We were selected because God knew we could handle it, that we individually and as a couple are strong enough. God knew we had the tools to pick up and continue to move forward. He knows those people who would not and could not move on. He knows it hurts but it will not end our lives. He knows that one day we will find the meaning in all this. He knows we are brave enough to face each day, to face our family and friends, to face the world. He knows we are smart enough to figure out His purpose for us and how this fits into His plan for our lives.

God picked us. This is not an accident. God makes no mistakes."

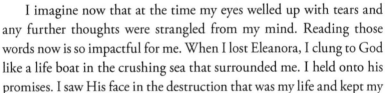

I imagine now that at the time my eyes welled up with tears and any further thoughts were strangled from my mind. Reading those words now is so impactful for me. When I lost Eleanora, I clung to God like a life boat in the crushing sea that surrounded me. I held onto his promises. I saw His face in the destruction that was my life and kept my eyes on Him. I look back and know I could not have done it without Him holding my hand and without His arms wrapped around me.

I lost my way when I found out I was having my first boy. I was convinced God no longer heard my prayers. I had pleaded with God to help save Eleanora and He stood by idly (keep in mind these are my thoughts at the time). Then I had prayed for months to have another baby girl, only to find out I was having a boy. I felt let down that He ignored everything that I felt was best for me.

It is difficult for others to understand this seemingly ungrateful reaction and mixed bag of emotions regarding my second child being a boy. After losing a baby, how could I even care if the next one was a boy or a girl? I had simply put all my faith in the idea that having another girl would help fill the void that was left when Eleanora went to heaven. I love my children dearly so don't get me wrong, but during that time period, I thought my heart would have healed with less jagged edges if I were to have another girl. This was the root of the anger and hurt I held onto for so long.

A friend of mine lost her daughter, Isabella, the same day I lost Eleanora. We met by pure accident after our daughters went to heaven. We were both in the hospital at the same time, our worlds crashing around us, completely unbeknownst to the other.

She had another daughter after Isabella. When Lily was about two years old, my friend texted me to say how bad she felt for me. She felt guilty that she ended up having the girl we both so desperately wanted and I ended up with two boys. It was so comforting to know she felt this way as I was often envious of her good fortune.

Now I know it is not good fortune, it is fate. She was meant to have Lily and I was meant to have my two boys. I may not understand God's plan, but I know I was meant to be their Mommy and they to be my children. There is no one else more suited for me than them and vice versa. God is good and He knows what he is doing.

Chapter 26

A Friendship from God

*Come back to the place of safety, all you prisoners who still have hope!
I promise this very day that I will repay two blessings for each of your
troubles.*

Zechariah 9:12 (NLT)

I met Isabella and Lily's mom by pure chance. A friend of Danielle's
looked up Eleanora's obituary on the funeral home page and noticed
two names of two little girls that had both died the same day. She told
Danielle who then told me.

Forgetting my own grief temporarily, I felt so much sympathy for this other family who was also suffering the loss of a child. I was surrounded by people who had experienced the loss of a child. My mom lost my eldest brother, Danielle lost her daughter, and my cousin lost her first daughter. Something in my gut told me this woman I'd never met was alone in her grief.

I found Isabella's name on the funeral page and reached out to the family. My email was sent in a letter to Isabella's family. Later, I found out that Isabella's dad, Dave, broke down in tears when he opened the letter and read its contents. Christina did the same. I was really surprised when I got an email from Christina after she received my letter.

Here are parts of Christina's first email, sent about a month after we lost our daughters:

Hi, this is Christina. You sent me and Dave a message about losing your baby. I'm truly sorry for loss :(I don't understand why these things happen! It just doesn't make any sense at all. I can't imagine taking home my baby and losing her 5 days later :(

But I do know all too well how you are feeling and there is nothing I can say to make you feel better. I actually lost our daughter on the first day of my last trimester. I was 27 weeks and she was born stillborn. I never got to hear her cry, I did however did get to hold her and now I have empty arms also :(

My doctor didn't catch that I had developed preeclampsia at my last prenatal visit. The day I lost her I was getting ready for work and noticed spotting and went to triage, it was a day that changed my life forever...

My health deteriorated within hours, blood pressure was through the roof and I had been told my baby girl did not have a heartbeat (she had been growing perfectly in every way up until then) and that I would have to deliver her. Literally the worst day of my life. I had her around 11pm that night after being induced. The hospital let us keep her in the room as long as we wanted, my sister took tons of pictures and we all held her. It was very surreal, like a dream almost. I never had that "awesome feeling" after delivery that moms get because I already knew she wasn't alive and I guess my brain processed it quickly...I still think about that day, everyday :/

Isabella was born with her cord around her neck two times, but the cause of her death according to the pathology report included that and also damage to the placenta due to my hypertension, but she was in perfect condition otherwise which breaks my heart :(

I'll pray for you and hope things get easier for you. Feel free to email me if you want to share your story, Dave may email you, I'm not sure though, he has been wanting to talk to people who have gone through this kind of situation.

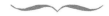

Christina was a lifeline for me throughout that summer and my next pregnancy. She was always there to text when I needed her. We shared a lot of bad days with each other. She was a gift sent straight from God. Although I had others in my life who had lost a baby, Christina's grief was as raw and fresh as my own. I needed the support of someone who was in my current situation. I didn't want to hear that things would get better because it didn't feel like that would ever be the case. She was just there to listen and to be a sounding board. It also felt great that I could fill that role for her too.

It turned out I was right that she didn't have anyone in her life who had experienced the loss of a child. She had been floating alone, but not anymore. Now we had each other. Through text messages, we were sad together, shed tears together, longed desperately for another baby together, charted our periods together, experienced the overwhelming frustration of my 49-day cycle together and finally celebrated the appearance of two lines on a home pregnancy test together.

No detail was left unshared. She was not only my cheerleader, encouraging me to test even when I thought it was too soon, but also my source of comfort when the test turned out to be negative. After eventually getting a positive test and telling Nick the good news, she was the next to find out that those two magical lines had at long last appeared.

We weathered all the highs and lows together. While she supported and encouraged me, I did the same for her. I listened to her frustration as it took her and Dave awhile longer to be ready to have another baby. I knew she was as desperate as I was to get pregnant again, but it wasn't until after I had Pierce that she conceived another child. Her hormone levels were really low at first which scared her, but she was pregnant. I was there for every worry and symptom she had throughout her pregnancy. Lily was born full term and healthy.

Right after Lily was born, I got pregnant with Everett and we went through that pregnancy together as well. I joked with Christina that she had to continue our tradition by getting pregnant again. She opted not to continue it.

God knew we needed each other through those times. When we met in person for the first time after being "pen pals" for a week or so, it was very cathartic for all of us. While Christina and I had each other, Dave really needed to vent and he felt most comfortable in a group of people who had all just lost their babies.

Now looking back, I see how life changing our friendship was and how God was truly looking out for all four of us. It is easier to see the blessings looking back. His hand was in the midst of it all. He was not ignoring our prayers or seeking vengeance on us. He was leading us all down different unexpected paths to bring us together to walk side by side through our grief and subsequent joys of three more healthy babies.

I hope you find a friend, relative, or neighbor to bond with after the loss of your child. I hope you are blessed like I was.

Chapter 27

Rainbow

So the Lord blessed Job in the second half of his life even more than in the beginning. For now he had 14,000 sheep, 6,000 camels, 1,000 teams of oxen, and 1,000 female donkeys. He also gave Job seven more sons and three more daughters. He named his first daughter Jemimah, the second Keziah, and the third Keren-happuch. In all the land no women were as lovely as the daughters of Job. And their father put them into his will along with their brothers.

Job 42:12-17 (NLT)

Job lived 140 years after that, living to see four generations of his children and grandchildren. Then he died, an old man who had lived a long, full life.

Babies born after a loss have a very special name: Rainbow Babies. I have two Rainbow Babies.

When I finished this book, I still felt like something was missing. It wasn't until I read the first chapter to Pierce that I knew just what it was. He asked me where his chapter was and to read it to him.

I have talked about the kids throughout the book. They are both so special to me. I raise them differently than other parents. I am more overprotective than other parents. They are my precious Rainbow Babies.

I was afraid the entire time I was pregnant with Pierce. I was hesitant to buy clothes or set up his room. I was afraid of losing him every day. I had a lot of contractions starting at 16 weeks and was put on bed rest when I was seven months pregnant.

When it was finally time for Pierce to come, labor and delivery were not easy. Pierce came into the world the way he has lived his life thus far - by the beat of his own drum.

After 30 hours of labor, it was decided we needed an emergency c-section. It came as no surprise to me that he was not descending as he should as I had been telling my doctor and the hospital staff that his head was not engaged like Eleanora's. When they opened me up, Pierce's head was in my hip. He was born at 10:06 p.m. on July 27. He was healthy and beautiful.

Everyone fell in love with him immediately. Before I got a chance to see him up close, the doctor told me he looked just like his sister. Words I hold close to my heart. When people see their pictures, they assume they were twins.

Pierce is special in his own right. He is very creative, intelligent, and funny. His mind works in fascinating ways. I hope he continues to show the world that being unique is not a negative thing. I believe he can change the world.

He is also special because he often gives us a glimpse of Eleanora. Maybe not in temperament, but in appearance and by "visiting" her in heaven. He is a rainbow baby in every sense of the word. He is a promise from God. He is a miracle. He wears the "Rainbow Baby" badge well. He will tell anyone about it and about his love for his big sister.

When it was time to prepare a room for Pierce, we weren't quite ready to paint Eleanora's purple walls decorated with bees, dragonflies, and a little green frog overlooking her changing table. So, we decided to give Pierce the third bedroom in our house. He has green walls with teddy bears in planes. We were afraid to decorate too much.

When we found out Everett was a boy, we knew we needed to change Eleanora's room to be Everett's. It was crushing. One day, when Pierce was about 18 months old, he and I went into Eleanora's room to pack away all of her clothes. I got a box and started moving all of her things from her dresser to the box. Tears streamed down my face with every outfit packed, with every lost dream stuffed into this box. Pierce looked at me and began to take all of Eleanora's things and return them to her dresser. Piece by piece he put them back in the drawers. I watched him stunned. When the last outfit was tucked in the drawer and the drawer was closed, he walked over to me, grabbed my hand with his chubby little hand and led me out of the room. He didn't have many words then, but I knew what he was saying, "Not today, Mommy. You aren't ready yet." I can still see the kindness and empathy in his little face. He was right. When it was the right time, he and I went back and he helped me pack everything up to make room for his little brother.

I was much more relaxed when I was pregnant with Everett. I had Pierce to distract me. I had Pierce to show me everything would be just fine. Everett's delivery was much easier than his older siblings. He came shooting out of me on the last push at 3:07 p.m. on May 29. When he was placed on my chest, I felt like our family was complete. He was the last piece to our family puzzle.

Before Everett was born, I didn't know how I could split my heart between three babies. I remember holding him as a newborn and falling so impossibly and deeply in love with him. It was magical.

My friend, Danielle, told me about her son's double spirit – that he has his sister's spirit in him. When she told me, I did not really understand. I didn't have kids then. Everett was about a year and a half when I saw the double in him. I believe he has his sister's spirit in him. He is as sweet as pie and oh so caring for his Mommy. He's also ornery and always keeps us on our toes.

These are my rainbow babies. They gave me hope again when I had none. They filled my broken heart with joy. While they have just one chapter in this book, they fill chapter after chapter in my life. They are not just Eleanora's brothers. They are their own books whose pages I am so blessed to read as they are written day by day.

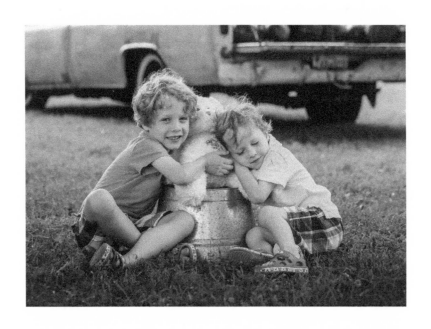

Chapter 28

My Hope is in You Alone

And we know that God causes everything to work together for the good of those who love God and are called according to his purpose for them.

Romans 8:28 (NLT)

The words to the MercyMe song "Even If" take me right back to the emergency room on June 22, 2011. I was pleading with God not to take my baby. I prayed on a loop. "Please God. Please don't take her. Please God. Please help her be okay." MercyMe echoes my prayer with these words:

"I know You're able and I know You can
Save through the fire with Your mighty hand...
I know the sorrow, and I know the hurt
Would all go away if You'd just say the word"

God did not answer my prayer the way I wanted that day. That does not mean, He did not answer my prayer. That does not mean He was not listening. I believe He answered it with words something like:

"It's easy to sing
When there's nothing to bring (you) down
But what will (you) say
When (you're) held to the flame
Like (you are) right now"

I ask you, what will you say to your Heavenly Father when you are held to the flame like you are right now? Will you let this horrific time pull you away? Will you believe the lies Satan is whispering in your ear? I hope not. I hope you rise above and let God fill you with the love and plans He has for you. Even though it may be hard, I hope this loss makes you a better and stronger you! I hope that even when God leaves mountains unmovable your hope is in Him alone.

Chapter 29

You Are Chosen

This excerpt is adapted from Erma Bombeck by Kerin Lee. I have slightly altered some of the content to reflect a conversation between a soon-to-be-angel-mommy and her pastor. It gives a very different view of being a parent to an angel baby.

Did you ever wonder how the mothers of angel babies are chosen? I asked my pastor and this is what he said.

"Somehow, I visualize God hovering over Earth, selecting His instruments for propagation with great care and deliberation. As He observes and instructs His angels to take notes in a giant ledger. Finally, He passes a name to an angel and picked you to have an angel baby."

"Why me? I am so happy."

"Exactly," my pastor says. "Could God give one of His precious angels to a mother who knows no laughter? That would be cruel."

"But do I have the patience to endure such hardship?"

"God doesn't want you to have too much patience, or you'll drown in a sea of self-pity and despair. Once the shock and resentment wear off, you'll handle it. God watched you today. You have that sense of self and independence so rare and so necessary in the mother of an angel. You see, the child He is going to give you lives in a world of its own. You will have to realize it lives in another world, and that's not going to be easy."

"But I don't think I even can live through this."

"No matter, God can fix that. You have just the right amount of selfishness."

"Selfishness?! Is that a virtue?"

"If you can't separate yourself from your angel baby occasionally, you will never survive. Yes, you are a woman whom God will bless with an angel less than perfect. You don't know it yet, but you will be envied. You will never take for granted a spoken word from anyone. You will never consider a minor step ordinary. You will never hear your angel say 'mama' for the first time, you will never be a witness to that miracle. God will permit you to see clearly the things He sees – ignorance, cruelty, prejudice – and allow you to rise above them. You will never be alone. God will be at your side every minute of every day of your life because you are doing His work as surely as you are here by my side."

Chapter 30

Thank You

I want to thank you as the reader for listening to my story and taking this walk with me. If you are a bereaved parent like me, you are on my mind and in my prayers. You are not alone. You are never alone. Even though the walk feels lonely, you have a crowd of supporters around you if you are brave enough to just lift your face. We may never meet. We may live thousands of miles away from each other. But know, I am here, walking with you. Our Heavenly Father is also always by your side. He knows you and He knows your very special baby. Keep the faith and the hope that you will one day be together again. Your baby is in heaven with my baby and all the other babies gone too soon.

Resources

Organizations –

- March of Dimes – The March for Babies walk is a great way to remember your baby and keep their memory alive. Find your local chapter www.marchofdimes.org

To donate to our team, go here: https://www.marchforbabies.org/EleanoraLynn

- Share – my local chapter does a Walk to Remember that has been very cathartic for my family. Find your local chapter www.nationalshare.org. They can also be found on social media.

Books -

"Lessons from a Rock Star: Rocked to the core while encountering God's supernatural peace, joy, hope and love" by Kristen Lopez

"Letting Go of Baby" and "What's Next?: A guide to dealing with grief after a loss" by Tamar Knibye

"Always Within; Grieving the Loss of Your Infant" by Melissa I. Eshleman

"Empty Cradle, Broken Heart, Revised Edition: Surviving the Death of Your Baby" by Deborah L. Davis

"Grieving the Child I Never Knew" by Kathe Wunnenberg

"The Courage to Grieve" by Judy Tatelbaum

"I Will Carry You" by Angie Smith

"Three Minus One: Stories of Parents' Love and Loss" by Sean Hanish

"Sunshine After the Storm: A Survival Guide for the Grieving Mother" by Alexa H. Bigwarfe

"Mommy, Please Don't Cry: There Are No Tears in Heaven" by Linda Deymaz

"I Carried an Angel" by Staci A. Luker

"Life Touches Life: A Mother's Story of Stillbirth and Healing" by Christiane Northrup M.D.

"Someone Came Before You" by Pat Schwiebert – a book for children

"My Baby Big Sister: A Book for Children Born Subsequent to a Pregnancy Loss" by Cathy Blanford

"A Guide for Fathers: When A Baby Dies" by Tim Nelson

"Love Mom: A Mother's Journey from Loss to Hope" by Cynthia Baseman

On the net -

After losing Eleanora, I joined the "Trying to Conceive After a Loss" group on www.thebump.com. This site has a ton of different types of groups. When I got pregnant I moved over to the "Pregnant after a Loss." I don't think these women understood how supportive they were. Even though I never posted anything other than an introduction, I knew I wasn't alone in my journey or in my fear of losing another baby.

There are also several groups or pages on Facebook that offer support. Here is one: https://www.facebook.com/iamamothertoanangel/

Another website with a lot of resources - https://www.irisremembers.com/

Find a group -

Admittedly, it took me awhile to find a group. I was involved with March of Dimes and Share. I was on the Bump forums. Everett was six months old before I found an "in real life" group. That group made a world of difference in my life. We were all moms with losses that were all so different, but we were all moms with a baby in heaven. I cried, shared my story, found healing, and honestly, never laughed so hard in the comfort of that group. Journey Angels ladies – you all are amazing women! I found my group at church, but that doesn't mean that is where you'll find your best fit. Don't go through this alone. If you can't find a group, start one. There is a need for it and you'll never regret it. My friend, Melissa, started Journey's Angels after losing her son Matthew. Later she and I started leading the group together. I hope all of the ladies got as much out of that group as I did.

Find a therapist -

There is no shame in seeking out help. This path is so difficult. It is so lonely and hard to navigate. I encourage you to at least try therapy and see if it works for you. It might help just to speak your child's name without any judgement or uncomfortable stares.

Things to bring peace:

- Molly Bears makes bears that weigh as much as your baby did. Inspired by her own story of loss, Bridget Crews, started making bears for her friends who had lost a child. This has turned into a wonderful organization. When I received my Eleanora Molly Bear, I could not stop crying. When I lifted my 7-pound 13-ounce pink bear out of the box, I couldn't let go. For the first time since June 22, 2011, it felt like I was holding my baby girl. I rocked that bear like she was real and the tears I cried were so healing. Our Molly Bear comes to our family pictures. The first year our photographer gave us a questioning look, but now she expects our Eleanora bear to come and even tells the kids to give their sister a hug while she photographs our whole family. You can find all the info to receive your own Molly Bear here: https://www. mollybears.org/.

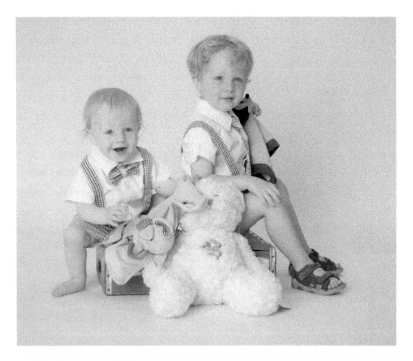

- Willow Tree also has several pieces to represent your angel baby or your time spent with your precious baby. My cousin, who lost her baby girl two years before Eleanora, sent me one of these beautiful pieces in the weeks after Eleanora went to heaven. These things bring me comfort and I hope they do the same for you. https://www.willowtree.com/

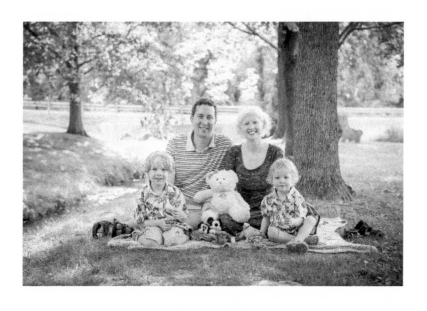

You adopted wings and flew away
so quietly one morning.
But to my side you often come
To remind me that you're never truly gone.
All our love,
Mommy, Daddy, Pierce & Everett

About the Author

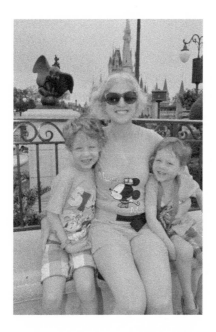

Natalie Scott is a mother of three beautiful children. She has been a writer for Easterseals for over a decade but has been writing for as long as she can remember. She has a story published in Chicken Soup for the Soul – The Magic of Mothers and Daughters and Chicken Soup for the Soul – for Mom with love. She started writing The Sun Will Rise after she lost her daughter, Eleanora. She has an adventurous spirit and loves to travel with her husband and children. They are all Disney fanatics!

CPSIA information can be obtained
at www.ICGtesting.com
Printed in the USA
BVHW082109040719
552613BV00002B/285/P